Zoku Shin Do®

The Art of
East Asian Foot Reflexology

Book One:
Japanese Foot Massage

D1718500

Zoku Shin Do®

The Art of East Asian Foot Reflexology

Book One: Japanese Foot Massage

Popular Edition compiled from
Zoku Shin Do, the Art of East Asian Foot Reflexology
Professional Edition
& Anma: The Art of Japanese Massage
Professional Edition

Mochizuki

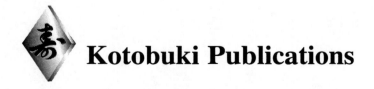
Kotobuki Publications

Zoku Shin Do®
The Art of East Asian Foot Reflexology
Book One: Japanese Foot Massage
Popular Edition

Published in the United States by

Kotobuki Publications
P.O. Box 19917
Boulder, CO   80308-2917

ISBN : 1-57615-010-0
Library of Congress Cataloging-in-Publication Data

NOTE TO THE READER:

All materials and instructions contained in this book require supervised training by a qualified professional. Authors, publisher, or Japanese Massage and Bodywork Institute are not responsible for the effects of the procedures contained in this book. All matters regarding your health require medical supervision and these materials are not a substitute for qualified care or treatment.

Printed in the United States

First Edition

5 ^{7} 6 ^{4}

Acknowledgements

In the process of creating this and other Zoku Shin Do books, I have many, many people to thank. This book would not have been possible without each person's unique contributions, both direct and indirect. I appreciate their support, and it is my hope that the readers of this book see the value of their contributions of positive energy.

I would like to thank my grandmother for sharing her knowledge and guidance with me, and for leading me to the study and practice of traditional Japanese medicine and massage. I thank my family members and ancestors who have practiced traditional medicine for over two centuries.

I also deeply appreciate my family, particularly my mother and father, who have always provided support.

Thanks to James Yule for his wonderful photographic contributions.

Thank you to Jeffrey Stevens and Kimbo Snyder for technical editing of the book.

A very special thank you to Mark Manton and Hilde Kraft of the Massage Therapy Institute of Colorado for their generous support of Zoku Shin Do and Japanese Massage education.

Also, my deepest appreciation goes out to all the staff and students of the various massage schools who have supported our ongoing education and have made our workshops possible.

Thanks to many of my friends who have helped in numerous ways, and the many people who have supported my practice over the years.

Production Staff

Special thanks to the following people and the many others who have been involved with this project over the years.

Inside	Editor-In-Chief	- Jeffrey Stevens
	Photography	- James Yule
	Models	- Cory Stephanson
	Text Editing	- John Siqveland
		- Kimbo Snyder
	Graphics	- Brian Mathews
	Japanese Calligraphy	- James Mochizuki
Cover	Design	- Brian Mathews
	Photography	- James Yule
	Model	- Cory Stephanson

FORWARD

Most people think a foot massage is just for the feet, but the effects of a foot massage are far-reaching. Foot massage can correct distortions in the feet in order to repair or relieve general structural imbalances. Foot massage is also used to balance corresponding reflecting internal organs through stimulation, and to reduce or eliminate many common ailments caused by living in modern society. In the fifteen years of my professional practice, I have integrated several forms of traditional Japanese bodywork and healing arts. Japanese foot massage and Zoku Shin Do (along with Anma) are undeniably my favorites. I admire these arts very much and I do not consider performing my daily treatments without them. After studying this book, I am certain that you will see a completely different way of understanding the feet and foot massage.

Massage, Anma, Shiatsu, and other forms of bodywork have been becoming more popular in recent years. You will find it both easy and beneficial to integrate Japanese foot massage into any modality of massage. Those of you who practice foot reflexology or perform pedicures will also find it easy to integrate Japanese foot massage into your practice. Japanese foot massage and Zoku Shin Do are unique and powerful forms of the healing arts. Its own history goes back over 5000 years, while being an independent form of foot reflexology for over 2000 years. Foot massage alone is one of the best massage techniques I have studied over the years, and I welcome this opportunity to share it with you.

Since I completed *ANMA: The Art of Japanese Massage* in the fall of 1995, I decided to compose both a Japanese facial massage and a Zoku Shin Do textbook in order to make these practices available to students outside of my classroom. The early stages for developing this book began in 1993. At that time, when I began teaching Zoku Shin Do, I was unable to find any textbooks which provided technical information and practical instructions for the application of those techniques needed to assist my teaching. If I was going to continue teaching I would have to develop a textbook that provided students with the much-needed information.

The Zoku Shin Do text was initially over 700 pages long and still only explained the basics (which have relatively complex theories, diagnoses and clinical information themselves). As I presented these early Zoku Shin Do texts in some of my classes, many students seemed overwhelmed by the amount of information. In the winter of 1995, I started teaching the foot massage portion of Zoku Shin Do separately as "Japanese foot massage". Many therapists found that these techniques were easy to understand and beneficial without being as complex asZoku Shin Do. In order to explain these techniques more clearly, many things have been modified over the years. Over 2500 photographs were taken in the process of developing this book. During the spring of 1997, with the contributions of many people, this book was finally completed and is now available to students outside of my classroom.

My main focus in developing this book has been to explain the techniques of Japanese foot massage as clearly and precisely as possible. In this popular edition, I have selected techniques that are the easiest for a layperson to learn. A few techniques are slightly more advanced, but these are nesessary techniques for an entire foot massage. In addition, most of the technical medical terminology (such as muscle and bone names) have been reduced to terms more easily understood by the layperson. This book should provide a better understanding of the foundations of Japanese foot massage, and should be beneficial for the layperson as well as for massage therapists and other health professionals.

Thanks again to everyone who believed and supported my work over the years. I would also like to thank you, the reader, for your support. I very much hope you enjoy this volume.

James Shogo Mochizuki
Spring, 1997

Contents

Chapter 9. Foot Stretching Techniques Without Lubrication

Chapter 10. Foot Stretching Techniques

Chapter 11. Japanese Foot Massage Techniques Lay on the Stomach Positions

Chapter 12. Afterward

Index

Chapter One

INTRODUCTION

An old Japabnese proverb says, "The foot is the gate of ten thousand different illnesses." This simply means that many illnesses begin in the feet. When I began studying Zoku Shin Do fifteen years ago, it did not make much sense to me. I had always thought the purpose of a foot massage was to provide good circulation and comfort. I never realized a foot massage could have such far-reaching effects. Over the years of practice, it started to make more sense as to how the foot was so closely connected to a person's health and how important the foot really is.

Most people do not recognize how closely the condition of the feet are related to their overall well-being. The feet are the foundation of the human physical structure, as well as the foundation of human health. It must be remembered that the entire weight of the body is supported by the small area of the feet. The foot is designed to support this weight for an extended period of time without pain or fatigue. The feet and legs support the pelvis, which in turn, supports the spine. Even a slight misalignment in the feet can cause spinal distortions which not only negatively effect posture, but the entire nervous system as well. Because the nervous system directly controls the function of the internal organs, a person's overall condition is directly linked to the health of the feet.

A solid foundation is necessary for the stablility of any construction. Likewise, the feet are the foundation of bodily health. The habits and demands of the modern lifestyle can distort the foot. Fashionable footwear, lack of exercise, and weight problems all strain and distort the feet. The feet require additional care to compensate for these stresses.

Zoku Shin Do (traditional East Asian foot reflexology) includes Japanese foot massage and Anma (Japanese massage) which are two of the best health care methods I know of for preventing and curing ailments in daily life. Japanese foot massage is easy for anyone to learn, and the layperson can start using and benefiting from it immediately. Unlike other forms of holistic medicine, such as acupuncture and chiropractic, Japanese foot massage does not require years of study before you can begin your practice. In addition, you can perform Japanese foot massage on yourself to improve your own health. You can apply Japanese foot massage anytime and anywhere, even in front of the television. It is not necessary to have a massage table, you can apply it while on the floor or in a reclining chair.

The roots of Zoku Shin Do go back to ancient China, and are over 5000 years old. Over 2000 years ago Ka Da changed to a form of reflexology, both for treating and diagnosing. Zoku Shin Do and foot massage techniques have been kept primarily in folk medicine for centuries, rather than in trade or professional practices, until now. Of course, there are many professional practioners of Zoku Shin Do and foot massage techniques, both in history and in modern days.

Full body massage is always wonderful to receive, but you might encounter conditions where it is not suitable to give full body massage. Many Zoku Shin Do reflexology techniques, along with Japanese foot massage, have been used throughout history in many circumstances between the 8th and 10th centuries. In Japan, a medical practioner was not allowed to touch the body of the female members of the Imperial or warrior classes. The hands and feet, and the neck and head areas, were the only places that were allowed to be touched, except under life-threatening condtions. The best practioners were chosen to work on them in these cases, but the practioners were only permitted touching of the hands and feet. Many illnesses had to be both diagnosed and cured through the hands and feet. For this reason, the Zoku Shin Do practioner was highly valued.

Another place where the Zoku Shin Do foot massage was used for centuries was in the inns in many villages of Japan. People would walk for miles traveling through Japan. When they entered the inn, many places would wash the travelers' feet and give massages. Some skillful practioners would diagnose health conditions through the feet. Zoku Shin Do practices of this type dwindled earlier this century, though a few places yet continue these traditions today.

Perhaps the reason Zoku Shin Do and foot massage techniques have been kept more often in folk medicine, rather than with medical professions, is because it is easy to learn and one of the best health care methods for a layperson in maintaining good health. It does not mean that either Japanese foot massage or Zoku Shin Do do not have professional qualities or healing value, but I believe that the best medicine always starts at home - where it has been for over 2000 years.

Zoku Shin Do and Japanese foot massage would have perished centuries ago if the technique did not produce healing results. With such a long tradition, Zoku Shin Do has much to offer our chaotic world. While many western approaches to the healing arts such as chiropractic and western massage are still in the developmental stages, Zoku Shin Do and many eastern healing arts have been established systems for over 2000 years with minor modifications each century.

East Asian medicine is generally designed to be preventative, rather than applied to the treatment of specific kinds of illness. Daily or weekly applications of simple foot massage can improve health and help to prevent many different illnesses, as well as improving physical and psychological health.

In this book, or in any of my books, I do not teach Kata (set routine). If I were to show a routine, it might help a beginner by giving examples of a routine to work, but it could create a bigger problem. Some students might start giving the same routine of the foot massage all the time. Everybody has differently shaped feet, physical conditions, sensitivities, and needs. There is no one routine that works for everybody. Foot massage must be carefully adjusted to suit each individual. Experience will aid your judgement in selecting the right massage techniques.

Traditionally, East Asian medicines are preventive and individualized medicines, and are not socialized such as western medicines. Assembly-line practices for massage should be avoided, although they can be better than not giving a massage at all.

After understanding the basics, it is best to improvise following your experiences and your intuitions. If I were an art teacher, I would not tell you what paint to use, or what to paint. I prefer to supply different colors to the art and ideas. You must paint the way you are inspired. If the object you choose to paint is an apple, it is your decision whether it is painted grey, purple, or square. I am offering techniques. It is your inspiration that must complete the picture.

It is important to create your own art and your own style of Japanese foot massage and Zoku Shin Do, it does not have to be done exactly as I do it. I encourage you to create your own routines and techniques. One of my philosophies of massage is that you can do anything you want, as long as you do not hurt yourself and you do not hurt other people. You must be very carfeul not to hurt yourself by over-extending while performing the massage. Start by developing common sense regarding what you should and should not do during massage.

My goal is to give fundamental ideas and inspire people. Part of the massage is creation and improvisation. One of the most important teachings of massage is to not be afraid, as long as you do not hurt others or yourself, you can massage any way you want.

In the western culture, the giving and receiving of massage is not traditional in daily life. Many people are uncomfortable with having their body touched by someone, especially with a full body massage. You might find foot massage an easier way to approach a person who never has been massaged before. It is an excellent way to introduce the benefits of massage.

Japanese foot massage and Zoku Shin Do are very unique and powerful healing arts. As I explained earlier, it is much more than just giving a foot massage. It improves health, as well as the structural balance of your body.

Japanese foot massage is very easy to learn with virtually no side effects. It is difficult to hurt someone with foot massage, unless it is done on purpose. As long as you apply general common sense, very little can go wrong. It is a very safe and effective method (though the foot stretching techniques explained in Chapter 10 might require cautious application).

Japanese foot massage is a wonderful skill to know. Daily practice and receiving of Japanese foot massage, along with proper exercise and diet, is an effective way to maintain optimum health, prevent ailments, and ensure physical, spiritual, and psychological health. Nowadays, nearly everyone has some minor physical complaints, which most of the time are not categorized as illnesses. Japanese foot massage can provide significant relief from daily stress, help make your daily life more pleasant, and improve your overall sense of well-being.

Chapter Two

WHAT IS JAPANESE FOOT MASSAGE?

What is Japanese foot massage? Japanese foot massage is unique. It is completely different from Western forms of massage such as Swedish massage, and East Asian forms of massage such as Shiatsu and Anma. Japanese foot massage utilizes the massaging techniques of Zoku Shin Do, which is the oldest known form of massage in foot reflexology.

During the development of Zoku Shin Do reflexology, especially over the last three thousand years, a unique and very effective method of foot massage techniques have been created. The purpose of these is to warm up the muscle, before you apply heavy pressure for reflexology, allowing it to enhance the effects of the reflexology.

It is not certain how much of foot massage was developed in China before entering Japan, and how much Japanese practitioners added and modified over the centuries. There is quite a difference between the Chinese, Taiwanese, and Japanese practitioners who practice Zoku Shin Do in modern times. There is also a difference between the techniques that are used to apply foot massage. The most often practiced techniques that I have studied in Japan from Zoku Shin Do, I have introduced here as Japanese foot massage. Yet, they all originated in ancient China, along with all of the other massage methods and medicines that originated in China.

Just the foot massage portion of Zoku Shin Do, without the concept of reflexology, has been introduced in this book as Japanese foot massage. Japanese foot massage does not require studying the very complex theory of diagnosis and techniques of Zoku Shin Do itself. Yet, it still is a very effective method to gently stimulate the feet, as well as all of the corresponding internal organs to prevent ailment.

Japanese foot massage utilizes the massage techniques of Zoku Shin Do which is the oldest known form of massage in foot reflexology. Its origin can be traced back at least 5,000 years and it might even go back as far as 10,000 years (refer to Chapter 3 for further explanation of the history of Zoku Shin Do). Japanese foot massage involves stroking, kneading and stretching to stimulate the feet in order that they become and remain healthy. Over many years and after many trials, healers learned which specific areas of the feet were best to manipulate in order to promote health.

Japanese foot massage techniques can combine any style of massage and bodywork and draw upon aspects from all East Asian healing arts. Japanese foot massage includes a variety of stroking techniques from the very fast and light applications to deep and slow stimulating techniques. These are combined together to reduce tensions and pains on the feet as well as to stimulate internal organs. The internal organs are stimulated by applying pressure and working through the various meridians and tsubo. This is beneficial in restoring overall health (For a complete discussion on meridian and tsubo theory please refer to chapter three).

During the fifth century, monks travelled from China to Japan bringing their religious and medical knowledge with them. Over many years, this knowledge disseminated throughout the countryside and began to be widely accepted.

Japanese foot massage is one of the oldest forms of massage in the world and the first form of massage recorded in textbook form that still exists today.

How do Japanese foot massage and Western foot massage differ?

Japanese foot massage is unique. It differs from the foot massage component of Swedish and other Western forms of massage. Even though all of the techniques of Japanese foot massage are derived from Anma, it has evolved into its own form independent of Anma, Shiatsu, and other East Asian based massage methods for working on the feet.

The biggest difference between Japanese foot massage and other techniques is the focus of the massage. The goal of Japanese foot massage is to improve the flow of Ki (human bio-energy), to improve circulation, to balance the internal organs and meridians, and to enhance one's overall health. With Western forms of massage, the focus is solely on comfort, relaxation, and circulation. Japanese foot massage and Zoku Shin Do are used to enhance or maintain the client's physical and psychological health and treat various health-related or structural ailments. Traditional Asian medical theory and diagnosis can be used to understand the condition of each client's health.

Another difference is the depth at which Japanese foot massage is applied. Practitioners of Western massage have traditionally been taught to perform massage smoothly without causing any discomfort, not to "dig in" if they feel an abnormality. Japanese foot massage differs in that its purpose is mainly therapeutic, not relaxant. When applied properly, Japanese foot massage should cause slight discomfort to the client when there are abnormalities in the client's muscles or structure. But, in the long run, the client will be able to benefit significantly from a good, firm, therapeutic foot massage. This does not mean you should apply the massage with all of your might. You must start gently and gradually add more pressure until you reach the therapeutic level.

Western massage often teaches the practitioner not to communicate with the client during the massage because it will be difficult for the client to relax. Communication with the client is an essential component of Japanese foot massage and Zoku Shin Do. Proper feedback is necessary for understanding the conditions of each indivdual client to ensure the quality of the treatment. To continue effectively working on a therapeutic level, it is very important to gather information from your client so that you understand the locations, sensations and levels of discomfort or pain.

Another difference between Japanese foot massage and other techniques is that they are very different in a technical sense. The speed and depth of Japanese foot massage techniques can encompass a wide range of applications. Some hand applications are light, smooth techniques which use very fast movement to warm the entire foot. Other applications are slow, deep-stimulating techniques that improve health and restore balance to the meridians. Some Japanese foot massage techniques are much more advanced than conventional massage techniques and require more practice in order to master. Japanese foot massage also requires very precise and complex finger movement which Western massage does not.

The Importance of the Feet

The stresses and habits of the modern lifestyle cause more foot strain than ever before. Some jobs necessitate extended periods of standing in a single position. Long working hours leave little time for exercise. Some shoes no longer provide adequate support for the feet and these shoes can cause distortions. Applied regularly, Japanese foot massage helps to counter some of these negative effects on the feet.

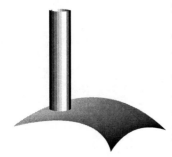

The foot is a unique structure. It supports the entire weight of the body in a very limited amount of space. It is made up of three different arches: the biggest arch is in the inside of the foot, the smaller arches are in the toes and outside of the foot. Imagine the foot as a curved triangle, touching the ground only at three points (see diagram to the left). It is crucial to have an even distribution of weight between these points to allow the foot to properly function.

When you take a step, one heel initially contacts the ground and body weight is gradually distributed all the way up to the toes. The ball of the foot remains on the ground and acts as a pivot as the toes push down and off the ground— propelling you forward. If you try to walk without using your toes, you will find that you need to compensate by lifting your knee and tightening your calves. This makes walking awkward, uncomfortable, and unnatural. Imagine the damage that would occur to your calves, knees and pelvis if you were to walk like this for years. This is they type of damage the toes sustain when a person wears improper footwear. The toes are as essential to the feet as the fingers are to the hand.

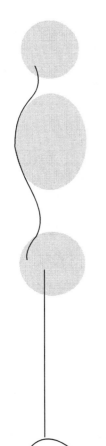

Many people force their feet into shoes that are tight and poorly designed. As a result, the big and small toes curve in toward the center of the foot. If the biggest and smallest toes are no longer sufficient to support the body, the entire body structure becomes distorted. This distortion is common in about 90% of women and 50% of men. This is because other regions of the body will be forced to compensate for the feet. When worn over a period of time, high-heel shoes will distort the natural curve of the foot, forcing the bone and muscular structure to shift to abnormal positions. This weakens the foot to the point where it can no longer support the body without fatigue and pain. The continuous pressure and daily stress put on the foot will result in a deterioration of full structural health.

Damaged arches are also becoming more common in many people. If the arch is damaged or flattened, the distribution of the weight over the foot's three main balancing points will shift. Over time, the foot will fail to sufficiently support the entire body weight. Even slight changes will result in feet which tire easily or unnecessary and cause harmful stress on the calf muscles which must compensate for the lack of foot support.

Early in this century, Dr. William Fitzgerald introduced Zone
Therapy foot reflexology in the United States. Shortly after this, several different European practicioners began introducing various other
methods of reflexology. In this century, there has been more scientif-
ic study about links between pressure points in the feet and various
health conditions than ever before in the West. In Asia, Zoku Shin
Do reflexology had been treating various forms of illness (even psychological conditions) 2000 years before Western medicine reached
Asia.

In Eastern Asia, the foot is traditionally known as the "barometer"
which reflects the condition of one's health. As I mentioned briefly
in the last chapter, traditional East Asian medicine has been using the
foot as an important source in a diagnostic method known as Kan Shi
Ho for over 5000 years. Many irregularities in the overall condition
of one's health appear in the feet.

An old Japanese adage literally states that "the sole of the foot is
another heart." Traditionally, it is believed that there are very close
links between the sole of the feet and the heart. In this model, the
sole of the foot is as essential for circulation as the heart. The heart
pumps blood throughout the body and the sole of the foot pumps the
blood back to the heart. In the old days people used to walk for
miles. If the foot was not properly taken care of, the rest of the body
was forced to work harder to compensate and the heart had to work
harder.

In Japan, practitioners (or even laypeople) are able to judge the overall condition of one's health by simply looking at the feet. The
underside of the feet should be a reddish-pink color. Dark pink or
grayish feet generally indicate a kidney or liver irregularity. If a person is healthy, the underside of the feet are full and firm. The underside of the feet of an unhealthy person are generally crumpled and
wrinkly. Exceptionally dry feet often indicate that a person will suffer from backaches, spinal and/or pelvis distortion. Other irregularities in health can also be "divined" from looking at the feet.

The foot is the foundation of human health and structure. Proper
care of the feet can improve your overall health as well as your pos-
tuire and structure.

Distortions of the Foot

There are a number of things that create foot distortion. Although distortions can be genetic in origin, lack of exercise and weight gain are more often causes. The largest single cause of foot distortion comes from shoes. There are many ways in which shoes affect the functioning of the feet.

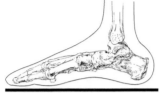

One type of shoe that is notorious for causing distortions is the raised heel or "high heel shoe". The raised heel causes an uneven distribution of weight among the three main supportive points on the foot. The job of supporting the majority of the body's weight falls on the minute outside corners of the balls of the big toes. When shoes are worn for long periods of time, bone constructions are positioned unnaturally, some ligaments and muscles are constantly overstretched and stress causes both big toes to distort inward. All the fascial tissue (tough connective tissue) is also stretched and distorted which often causes surface pains.

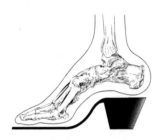

High heels were developed in conjunction with the tight corset and large, frilly dresses during the seventeenth and eighteenth centuries in France. At that time, men thought women looked more attractive in high heels because the shoes made them slightly taller and made their hips thrust outward more. The legs and feet suffered and walking was made awkward, but the men still found the appearance to be "cute." This practice is still popular throughout the world even though it is a leading hidden cause of many health problems.

High heels do not only distort the feet, however. They cause distortions throughout the entire structure of the body. Wearing them causes extra tension on all muscles from the calves to the lower back which, in turn, causes the pelvis to rotate forward and outward. This makes the lower back move forward and causes the hips to jut out backwards. This also causes the legs to rotate inwards which can cause a person to be pigeon-toed. Wearing high heel shoes for long periods of time also restricts and weakens the Achillies' tendon. The pelvis and legs are forced to compensate as a result of this. Many people who suffer from lower back pains can attribute the problem to improper footwear.

Another problem with many shoes, especially women's footwear, is that the toe of the shoe is so narrow that the biggest and smallest toes of the feet become cramped and inwardly distorted. When these shoes are worn for prolonged periods of time, the toes lose their natural range of motion. The abductive (closing inward) and adductive (spreading outward) movements are especially impaired.

In addition, some shoes do not provide enough structural support to the arches and many peoples' arches are completely destroyed because of this. Neglecting to wear sensible and quality footwear costs some people the ability to stand for long periods of time without fatigue. Although people may claim that they have suffered from problems with their arches all of their lives, it must be remembered that human beings are born without arches. Arches develop during one's first five years. This is why wearing shoes in the earliest formative stages of life can hinder the development of proper foot structure.

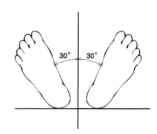

Shoes also reduce stimulation to the bottom of the feet. Obviously, a person can not go everywhere with bare feet in today's society, but proper stimulation on the bottom of the feet is very important for maintaining the health of internal organs. A recent study in Japan has shown that children who do not wear shoes generally stay healthier, have better brain development and develop better memorization skills than children who do wear shoes. Structural problems are also found less frequently in children who do not wear shoes.

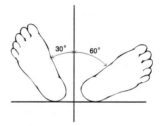

In Western culture, most people wear shoes from the time they wake up until they go to sleep. In Japan, people limit the amount of time they spend wearing shoes by only wearing them when they go outside. This increases the amount of foot stimulation and decreases the amount of time the natural contours of the foot are restricted.

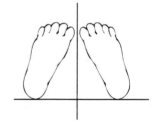

In the past, shoes were created to fit each individual. Modern production methods create shoes of prefixed sizes. Finding shoes with exactly the proper fit takes time and effort. It may be that none of the prefixed sizes available will properly fit the contours of your feet. Often, people are not willing to spend enough time looking for shoes with the best fit. Instead, they look for shoes based on fashion or price. These shoes may look better or cost less, but in choosing them the health of your feet and body may be compromised.

Good shoes generally cost more, but they are a good investment. Expensive shoes generally last much longer than cheaply made ones. Although cheaper shoes may look the same, you may find that they begin to fall apart in the time it takes to break them in because they do not properly support the feet. It is also better to have a few pairs of well-fitting shoes than to have many different types of shoes. Changing into different shoes every day can cause foot strain and discomfort.

It is very important to select proper footwear that will prevent and reduce foot distortion. Often, this in itself will reduce or eliminate many structural problems and problems relating to structure such as shoulder tension or head aches. Generally the best footwear, such as some types of sandals, will restrict the foot very little. It essential that footwear fits well, supports the arches adequately and allows full lateral movement in the toes.

Why is Japanese Foot Massage Important?

Frequent applications of Japanese foot massage have many benefits. These include repairing distortions in the feet, stimulating tsubo and internal organs and improving one's overall health condition. This process is relatively slow, however. Restoration time depends on how severe the foot distortion is and how often it is treated. Of course, foot structure will not be restored in a few days. Depending on its severity, it may take up to several years to repair the distortions.

Repairing distortions in the feet not only improves the structure of the foot itself, but the body's entire structure and alignment. As proper foot alignment is restored, any distortions in the pelvis and spine which may have been caused by imbalances in the feet will gradually correct themselves. Similarly, Japanese foot massage can be used to reduce many structurally related problems caused by high body tension such as lower back ache, shoulder and neck tension, and headaches. Foot massage also restores the arch which makes it much less tiring to stand up for long periods of time.

Japanese foot massage also promotes proper blood flow to the feet. As the human system converts air and food to get energy, it releases unwanted gas and toxins through blood vessels. These are divided into three catagories: veins, capillaries and arteries. Arteries carry oxygen througout the body to the capillaries. Capillaries bring oxygen to individual cells. Here, oxygen is exchanged for carbon dioxide and waste toxins. Veins then bring the waste products to organs which will expell them from the body. Often, unwanted toxins clog up capillaries. Most of the capillaries are less than one-hundredth the diameter of a human hair. If toxins clog blood flow in the capillaries, red blood cells can no longer provide oxygen and nutrients to indivdual cells. Toxins will then stagnate there. When blood vessels become clogged the nerve and lymphatic systems fail to function at peak level. Smaller areas of the body (such as the feet and hands) retain toxins longer than usual. Because they are continually in motion, the hands release toxins more quickly than the feet. Foot massage detoxifies the feet by freeing blood flow in the capillaries.

Japanese foot massage loosens tight or cramped muscles, ligaments and bones in the feet and ankles. It also helps to prevent further health problems from arising.

Japanese foot massage stimulates the internal organs which are reflected in the feet. Unlike Zoku Shin Do or other forms of reflexology, Japanese foot massage is not used to treat specific areas of the feet or specific health problems through stimulations. Yet, mild stimulations over each entire foot will stimulate the internal organs evenly to restore and enhance one's overall health.

Japanese foot massage also uses tsubo and meridians to balance the energy flow of the internal organs to enhance the health and prevent illness. The feet contain very important tsubo. Tsubo are points on the body that connect meridians. Meridians are pathways along which Ki (lifeforce energy) runs throughout the body. Kei Ketsu (tsubo on the meridians) are directly connected to individual internal organs and support their functioning. Sei Ketsu ("well" points, as in a "water well") are also located on the feet. These are among the most important points on the meridians that maintain and restore health.

Tsubo called Zoku Shin literally translate as "heart of the feet." These are known as "the most important points of all points" or "the points which govern and affect the one hundred meridians and one thousand tsubo on the body." Although these points are located on the bottom of the foot, they do not belong to any one meridian.

Very important meridians run into the feet. Proper functioning of kidneys, liver and spleen meridians are essential for maintenance and restoration of health. The foot is a very important part of proper meridian balance and functioning because it is the transition area between yin and yang meridians. Improving the connection between meridians improves the balance of the meridians which, in turn, leads to one's balanced health.

The foot itself is so closely connected with internal organs and meridians that you can treat most imbalances directly through the feet.

Japanese foot massage is thus important in three ways. Firstly, it can be used to diagnose problems in the feet and problems throughout the body caused by foot distortions. Secondly, Japanese foot massage can be used to treat and gradually repair structural damage which has been done. Thirdly, regular applications maintain the health of the feet and body.

Japanese foot massage is very easy for most people to learn and its benefits can be noticed instantly. You do not need to be a massage therapist to understand it, and it does not take years of study before you will be able to practice. Learning and applying even a few techniques will be beneficial. Japanese foot massage is very safe even for beginners to apply, and unlike other forms of medicine, Japanese foot massage has no side effects. Information about East Asian concepts such as meridians and tsubo have been listed in this book for interested readers. Although it may be helpful to be familiar with these concepts, it is not absolutely necessary to understand them in order to give and receive the benefits of Japanese foot massage.

Japanese foot massage can also help to restore the balance of emotions in conjunction with balancing the internal organs. Probably the greatest difference between Western and Eastern medicines is that physical and psychological conditions are separated in the West. In traditional East Asian medicine, the physical directly affects the psychological and vice versa. For example, strong, negative emotions can adversely effect the internal organs, just as a negative condition of the internal organs can produce psychological difficulties.

The condition of the emotions is closely related to daily health maintenance. In the traditional East Asian medicine, both physical and psychological components are taken into consideration when a person's overall health is evaluated.

Internal organ balance and emotional balance are interrelated. Emotional imbalance can be improved by treating the internal organs and meridians of the physical body (through Shiatsu, Anma, acupuncture or mind-body exercises like yoga or tai chi). Internal organ illness or imbalance can be restored by working on the emotions through practices such as meditation.

In The Yellow Emperor's Classic of Internal Medicine, the 2500 year-old text of Chinese medicine, the Emperor asks the Master how people can prevent illness. The Master answers, "As long as one's five internal elements (emotions) are completely balanced, one has perfect resistance to any outside illnesses." The Five Element theory is commonly used to balance the five corresponding emotions when dealing with psychological matters.

Traditionally, the five emotions are: sadness, fear, anger, happiness and worry. Experiencing these states of mind excessively or frequently can harm the health of the internal organs. Excessive emotions can be caused by internal organ imbalance, as well as causing internal organ imbalance.

A person can experience many emotions at one time. One emotion can affect another. More than two emotions can disturb each other.

The relationship between the physical and psychological must be recognized in order to determine the cause of a condition. When dealing with emotional issues, it is very important to be aware that these can be sensitive subjects for some people. Your character and rapport with your client can be either helpful or harmful. I suggest that you do not try to bring forth your client's emotional issues, but instead, be supportive if they are working through difficult issues.

Japanese foot massage is also a great method for improving relationships. In today's busy world, spending relaxing time together is
becoming more and more rare. Couples, friends, or families can use
Japanese foot massage to cultivate tenderness, intimacy, and a sense
of caring.

Chapter Three
ZOKU SHIN DO AND
JAPANESE FOOT MASSAGE

What is Zoku Shin Do?

Zoku Shin Do (also Soku Shin Do in Japanese; Zhak She Dao in Chinese) is probably the oldest known and recorded form of foot reflexology. Its history can be traced back to ancient China over 5000 years ago. Zoku literally means "feet" (the Japanese term for foot includes the foot, ankle, and leg). Shin means "heart" (or often "center" or "core"— the most important part of something). Do means "way"; it also indicates the entire art or discipline of an art.

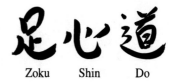

Zoku Shin Do is very rich in therapeutic value. It takes years of practice to master because it requires a deep understanding of East Asian medical theory, meridians, and tsubo. An essential part of Zoku Shin Do treatment is that one must first be able to assess conditions using pulse, abdominal, and other diagnostic methods, not just through foot diagnosis. All concepts in East Asian medicine — tsubo, meridians, internal organ reflections, and meridian reflections — require more intensive study in order to fully understand and perform Zoku Shin Do. An in-depth study of meridians and tsubo can take years.

Zoku Shin Do has its own unique set of foot massage techniques which are used to "warm up" the feet. These are used to stimulate the entire foot, to maintain health, and to prevent illness. These techniques are easy to learn and do not require an understanding of any concepts of diagnosis, yet they still comprise a very effective form of foot massage. In this book, I will introduce these massage techniques separately as "Japanese foot massage".

A Brief History of Zoku Shin Do

Zoku Shin Do is probably the oldest form of foot reflexology and can be traced back over 5000 years to ancient China. The oldest records referring to it are from the time of the Yellow Emperor (Haung Ti) where it is called Kan Shi Ho which translates as the "Foot Diagnosis Method". The oldest reference to Zoku Shin Do dates back approximately 2000 years ago to the Han Dynasty.

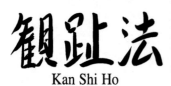

Kan Shi Ho

Zoku Shin Do was introduced by Ka Da, a well known doctor, as an independent medical system and taught to many health practitioners. His students carried on Zoku Shin Do practices which later gave rise to variations of the original form. Most were kept secret and passed down through generations of a family or community. For the last 2000 years Zoku Shin Do has survived in China as "folk medicine" (as opposed to the more traditional acupuncture or herbology).

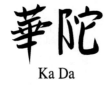

Ka Da

Another theory supposes that Zoku Shin Do originated in Nepal or India as a part of Buddha's teaching. A foot reflexology chart was created during Buddha's lifetime and was supposedly taught by him. Shortly after his death, it was carved into stones inscribed with other aspects of his teaching. These became the primary objects of worship for Buddha's followers until the commonly known Buddha figure was created several hundred years later. When Buddhism moved into China with the reflexology chart as its primary symbol, Ka Da combined it with native medical concepts to create Zoku Shin Do. Over the years, Zoku Shin Do has developed from primarily a foot diagnosis method to incorporating meridians (Keiraku), tsubo (acupoints), and diagnosis to become an inclusive therapy.

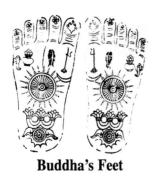

Buddha's Feet
Over 1600 years old,
stone carved
Yaku Shi Temple, Nara Japan

It is most likely that Zoku Shin Do entered Japan during the fifth century A.D. either directly from China or through Korea. We can only speculate as to when it actually arrived, however, because China and Japan have rarely been on friendly terms in the last 1500 years, and the earliest trace found in Japanese records is from the eighth century.

Foot massage techniques were added to Zoku Shin Do's reflexology methods approximately 2500 - 3000 years ago. All foot massage techniques originated in and were modified from Anma. These foot massage techniques underwent further modifications during the fourteenth through eighteenth centuries in Japan. During this time they became substantially different from the techniques used by practitioners in other Asian countries.

In modern times, Zoku Shin Do is practiced widely throughout East Asia. Each practitioner understands and applies Zoku Shin Do in a slightly different manner. Differences in the practice of Zoku Shin Do are especially apparent between Japanese and Chinese practitioners.

Zoku Shin Do Treatment

Unlike Japanese foot massage, Zoku Shin Do is generally used to treat specific conditions after diagnosing a client. Zoku Shin Do is divided into five major treatment methods. Each method has unique characteristics and offers its own advantages for treating different conditions. For example, a general foot massage will work best for someone who has a difficult time relaxing into the treatment. However, if someone suffers from a specific complaint, such as headaches or constipation, working with tsubo and internal organ reflections will treat those conditions more effectively. Although application of a single Zoku Shin Do technique is benevicial, it is always best to combine as many of them as possible to provide the best treatment.

Foot Massage - This portion of a treatment is used to relax the client. This will loosen muscles, allowing you to perform the remaining stages of the treatment with less difficulty and more effectiveness. Even performed independently of the other methods, this is an effective treatment for generally stimulating the entire foot and promoting better health. Chapters Five through Ten of this book are dedicated to introducing its many applications.

Tsubo - This refers to "acupoints". This part of Zoku Shin Do is the application of pressure to the tsubo on the feet, ankles, and sometimes the lower legs. Pressure may be applied to either tsubo on the meridians or to the Ki Ketsu (extraordinary points). These points are chosen based on the practitioner's experience in treating the diagnosed condition of the client. You will find a detailed explanation of tsubo on page 31.

Keiraku - Keiraku refers to meridians (see p 30). This procedure involves stroking the meridians to create or maintain proper Ki flow in the feet or legs. Stroking in different directions is used to tonify or sedate a meridian depending on what has been deemed necessary through diagnosis (see p 29 - 30).

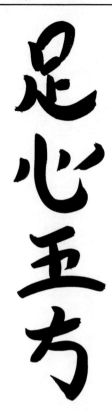

Internal Organ Reflection - By working the area of the foot where a specific organ reflects, the practitioner can stimulate a particular organ which is irregular. Organ reflection is outlined on page 42.

Meridian Reflection - Similar to organ reflection, meridian reflection attempts to stimulate a meridian by stroking its reflection on the body. Its purpose is to restore health and balance by tonifying or sedating particular reflecting meridians. Unlike Keraku or tsubo, using reflections can provide easy access to the Lung, Large Intestine, Heart, Small Intestines, Shin Po, and San Sho meridians that do not run through the feet. Please refer to page 43 for further explanation.

East Asian View of Health

There is a distinct cultural difference between the Eastern and Western views of health and health care. To practice Japanese foot massage or East Asian medicine, it is important to have a rudimentary understanding of the Asian concept of health.

In the West, people tend to rely on the diagnosis of a physician to define illness. A person may recognize being "in pain", "out of sorts", or "under the weather", but it is the physician who ultimately decides if the subject is functional or needs healing or curing. Treatment does not begin until a person has been officially diagnosed as "ill".

In East Asia, treatment is applied much earlier in the health care process. East Asian medical providers emphasize early diagnosis and prevention. Once noticeable symptoms appear, an illness is considered very advanced in Asian medicine. The objective of East Asian medicine is to diagnose illness in its early stages before symptoms appear. The thinking behind this is that treatment and recovery are easier and faster and the spread of disease is minimized.

In the West, little effort is made to strengthen the body before disease sets in. Once a person is officially ill, a rapid recovery or a "miracle cure" is sought. The hope or expectation that a physician will make these things available to them leads people to neglect health care on a day-to-day basis. Generally, this leads to an over-reliance on doctors and other medical practitioners.

In East Asia, the majority of people trust the ancient ways because of their rich historical and cultural tradition. In the United States, there are few traditional methods of healing based on time-tested remedies. Those that do exist, such as folk medicine, are often treated with suspicion.

Westerners generally wish for perfect health, an ideal that the wide majority of people cannot possibly attain. East Asian people do not believe in such a thing as "perfect health". It is simply accepted that people have irregularities and genetic differences. Each person must constantly negotiate well-being within the boundaries of personal health. In Asia, trying to achieve balanced health is the objective. Westerners tend to value the "instant cure" more than the efforts to gradually improve personal health.

It could also be argued that the Eastern view of health is more holistic than the Western view. For example, connections between the functions of the internal organs and the psychological health of people are rarely made in the West, but these are fundamental principles of East Asian medicine.

Ki

Ki is the Japanese spelling of the Chinese "Qi" (pronounced chi) which means "universal energy". Ki is very connected to everyday affairs in Japan. For example, people will ask, "How is your Ki today?" rather than "How are you?". In addition, disease is described as an illness of Ki (Byo Ki). According to traditional Tao theory, there are three different types of Ki energy which affect everything in the universe: Ten Ki, Ji Ki and Jin Ki.

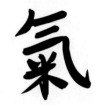

Ki - Universal Energy

"Ten" means "heaven" or "sky" and Ten Ki is the Ki which emanates from everything above ground level. The conditions of the sun, moon, sky, clouds, humidity and other aspects of the weather affect people just like life on the ground does. Notice how depressed some people can get after several cloudy, overcast days. Not enough rain (Ten Ki) causes a drought (Ji Ki) which will eventually affect peoples' internal organs (Jin Ki).

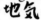

"Ji" means ground and Ji Ki is the Ki which comes from the ground. Ji Ki controls such things as soil, earthquakes, minerals, groundwater and heat from the earth's core. The condition of Ji Ki is affected by Ten Ki, but not by Jin Ki. Conversely, Ji Ki affects Jin Ki but not Ten Ki.

人気

Jin Ki is human Ki or "lifeforce energy". Jin Ki has no effect on Ten Ki or Ji Ki, but is affected by both. Therefore, the condition of the environment and nature is very important to human life.

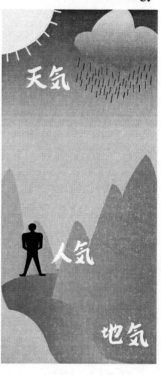

Zo Fu, Internal Organs and Zoku Shin Do

Zo Fu means internal organs in Japanese. There are five Zo Organs and six Fu Organs. Zo organs are the Yin organs— the lungs, heart, kidneys, liver and spleen. Fu organs are the Yang organs— the small intestines, large intestine, stomach, gall bladder, bladder and San Sho. The primary function of the Fu organs is to support the Zo organs. Eastern and Western medical thought systems understand the functions of the internal organs in completely different ways.

	Metal	Earth	Fire	Water	Wood
Zo Organ	**Lung**	**Spleen**	**Heart**	**Kidney**	**Liver**
Organ Function	• Conditions the *Ki Ketsu* (Ki and Blood) • Intakes Air (Heaven) Ki which later combines with Food Ki to become Original Ki • Distributes *Yang Ki* throughout the body	• Governs liquid and fluid movement • Distributes Food Essence throughout the body • Regulates menstruation	• Master organ, governs all other internal organs • Controls the spirit • Governs the *Ketsu* (Blood) circulation throughout the body	• Stores *Sei* • Distributes *Sei* to all internal organs as they need it • Governs hormonal levels and functioning, especially the growth process	• Governs Brain functions • Stores and regulates *Ketsu* • Governs musculoskelatal conditions
Fu Organ	**Large Intestine**	**Stomach**	**Small Intestine**	**Bladder**	**Gall Bladder**
Organ Function	• Supports Lung functions • Accepts waste from Small Intestine; separates liquid from solid • Eliminates solid waste; sends liquid to Bladder • Holds Primary Ki	• Supports Spleen functions • Examines, accepts and digests food • Converts food to *Sei* (nutrition) and waste by fermentation	• Supports Heart functions • Receives predigested food from the stomach and separates *Sei* (nutrition) from waste; sends Sei to Spleen and waste to Bladder and Large Intestine • Store and hold primary Ki	• Supports Kidney functions • Governs liquid and fluid levels in the body and eliminates excess amounts • Eliminates liquid waste from the Small and Large Intestines	• Supports Liver functions • Governs decision-making process • Stores *Tan Ju* (the very pure liquid of the gall bladder)

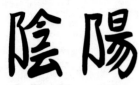

In Yo - Yin and Yang

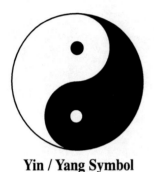

Yin / Yang Symbol

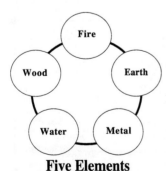

Go Gyo Setsu
- Five Elements Theory

Yin / Yang and the Five Elements Theory

Most people recognize the symbol of Yin and Yang. The concept of Yin and Yang is basically about balance between opposites and continual transformation. This concept is essential for understanding and practicing Zoku Shin Do as well as traditional East Asian medicine. Traditional East Asian medicine is all about balance. A person's health is directly related to how well-balanced that person is.

All traditional Japanese medicine is based upon the Taoist concept of opposites (Yin-Yang theory) and/or the Five Elements theory. In the Nei Ching it is said "the universe is an oscillation between the ebb and flow of the forces of Yin and Yan", which reflects the essential notion that all phenomena arise from the interplay of these two components. A common misunderstanding about Yin-Yang theory is that Yang is good and Yin is bad. Neither is any better or worse than the other; both are equally important aspects of the whole. Without understanding that which is negative, one cannot understand that which is positive. Because they drive each other, these two opposite aspects must be balanced to function properly . The Yin-Yang is not a judgemental philosophy of better or worse, it is a way of balance.

In traditional East Asian medical theory, Yin is often considered more important (not "better") than Yang. The purpose of Yang is to support Yin. The main function of Yang organs is to support Yin organs of the same elements; likewise, the main function of the Yang meridians is to support the functions of the Yin meridians of the same element. There is no absolute Yin or Yang; this is why each is shown containing a portion of each other. A black circle inside the white and a white circle inside the black illustrates that all Yin contains some Yang and vice versa. For example, you cannot get absolute darkness (Yin), nor can you get absolute brightness (Yang); darkness contains some brightness, just as brightness contains some darkness.

The Yin-Yang and Five Elements theories developed at separate times and places. It is commonly understood that the Yin-Yang theory developed first and is much older than the Five Elements Theory. In the Five Element theory, as in Yin-Yang theory, it is most important to keep each element harmoniously balanced with the others.

In the Five Elements theory, all things—time, seasons, directions, animals, planets, smells, etc., as well as internal organs—belong to one of five categories. The combination of the Yin-Yang and Five Elements theories make up the foundation of Japanese acupuncture and bodywork. This combination of theories originated in China and can be traced to the Chou Dynasty (1100 - 771 B.C.). It is believed to have entered Japan in the fifth century. Today, it is one of the distinct properties of Japanese bodywork and acupuncture.

**Five Elements
Mutual Position**

The mutual or beginning position of the Five Elements is shown at the bottom of the opposite page. In the diagram, the Five Elements balance harmoniously, maintaining a mutual relationship. This position describes perfect balance in nature, and from the medical perspective, in the internal organs. No one part interferes with the others, indicating perfectly balanced physical and psychological health. This combination of placement and balance creates the ideal state.

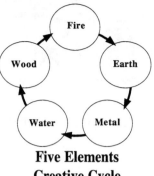

Five Elements Creative Cycle

The creative cycle represents the natural phenomenon of regeneration or creation. One element acts as creator and creates the next element in the clockwise cycle. For example, Water is necessary for creation of Wood, and Wood is necessary for Fire. This movement is also commonly used for Ho (tonification, see p. 27). If one element is depleted, another should support its creator element in order to tonify the element that has been depleted. This is also called the Mother-Son Law. For example, if the heart is depleted, its mother element (the liver) should be tonified (see diagram at lower right).

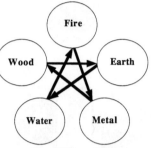

Five Elements Destructive Cycle

The destructive cycle represents the natural phenomenon of destruction or the control of one element over another. One element can be a destroyer and another element can be destroyed. For example, Water can destroy Fire and Metal can destroy Wood. This movement is also commonly used for Sha or sedation (see p. 27) meaning that if one element is too strong, it can be suppressed by its destructor element. This is recognized as the destroyer controlling the destroyed element.

The combination of the Yin-Yang and Five Elements theories shown here is commonly used in traditional Japanese Medicine as well as in East Asian medicine. Ten internal organs are placed into relationships between Yin and Yang, and among the Five Elements.

One additional purpose of Zoku Shin Do is to balance the Ki among the ten different internal organs. It can be very complex to address ten internal organs at once. It is more effective and less complex to balance first the Yin and Yang in each individual element, then to balance between the Five Elements.

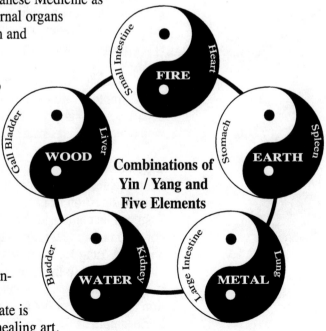

Combinations of Yin / Yang and Five Elements

These relationships illustrate the balance of the internal organs—the ideal sought by those who use Zoku Shin Do, traditional Japanese, and East Asian medicine. Understanding how these organs interrelate is critical when practicing any East Asian healing art.

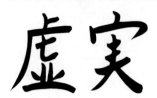

Kyo Jitsu
- Depleted and Excessive

Normal

Kyo
(Depleted)

Jitsu
(Excessive)

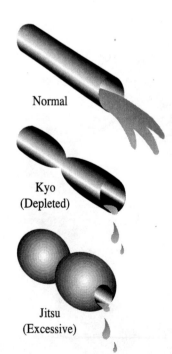

Normal

Kyo
(Depleted)

Jitsu
(Excessive)

Kyo (depleted) and Jitsu (excessive)

Kyo and Jitsu are terms used to describe the condition of each meridian's Ki flow for professional application of traditional East Asian medicine. The common English translations of Kyo and Jitsu are, respectively, 'depleted' and 'excessive'. In Chinese, they are pronounced as Hsu (Kyo) and Hsih (Jitsu). Traditional East Asian medicine does not name diseases or illness in the same way Western medicine does. Traditional East Asian medicine uses descriptions such as Lung Kyo and Spleen Jitsu to name an illness or condition. Western medicine requires a symptom before a diagnosis. In traditional East Asian medicine, conditions can be diagnosed long before noticeable symptoms appear.

Kyo and Jitsu describe the stagnation of Ki (energy flow). Either too little or too much Ki flow can cause stagnation. Quantity is not quality: too much energy flow can be just as damaging to the physical and psychological makeup as too little Ki flow.

Even a beginner should be able to assess whether a meridian is regular or irregular. Determining Kyo or Jitsu, however, is considered one of the most difficult skills to master in traditional East Asian medicine. Do not be discouraged by this— it takes a lot of practice to determine whether a condition is Kyo or Jitsu. If you keep practicing and developing these skills, you will soon be able to make an accurate diagnosis.

Kyo, the condition of depletion, translates as "lies", "untruths" or "superficial". The Ki flow is disturbed because not enough energy is going through the meridian. Kyo symptoms are usually not obvious, they are often hidden and must be sought out. An informed diagnosis is generally necessary to discover the Kyo symptoms.

Jitsu, the condition of excess, translates as "real", "exists" or "truths". Jitsu symptoms are more obvious than Kyo symptoms and are often discovered by simply listening to the client's complaints. These would include things such as heat, pain, aches or other obvious ailments.

Chronic conditions are typically Kyo, while acute conditions are typically Jitsu. For example, chronic stomach weakness is Kyo and acute indigestion or pain in the stomach region is Jitsu. Kyo and Jitsu can be combined with the Yin and Yang theory to describe a condition more precisely. There are four conditions of Kyo and Jitsu: Yin Kyo, Yang Kyo, Yin Jitsu and Yang Jitsu. Yin and Yang are closely related to the temperature of particular regions of the body, meridians and organs. A cold area generally indicates a Yin condition and a warm or hot area generally indicates a Yang condition. For example, if the liver is cold and depleted, it is a Yang Kyo condition and should be treated as such.

Ho (tonification) and Sha (sedation)

Ho and Sha are professional terms used only in Zoku Shin Do, Keiraku, Shiatsu, and East Asian medicine. They are used after the diagnosis to determine the condition of each of the twelve meridians (see pp. 30-31). Diagnosis determines whether one should tonify or sedate the meridian in order to balance it.

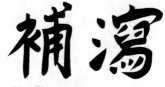

Ho Sha
- Tonification and Sedation

Ho is a Japanese name for "tonification" or "supporting". In the context of East Asian medicine, it means to tonify or raise the Kyo (depleted) condition. When one meridian is too weak, the creative cycle or Mother-Son law tells us that we need to support the creator or mother. For example, if the lung is Kyo, we should tonify (support) the mother— in this case the spleen.

Sha is the Japanese name for "throwing away" or "taking out". In the context of East Asian medicine, Sha means sedation or quieting a condition which is Jitsu (excess). When you find that one meridian is too strong, remember the destructive cycle of the five elements. Sedate the oppressor and you will sedate the meridian as well. For example, if the spleen is Jitsu or too strong, you could sedate the liver to calm the spleen.

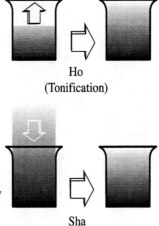

Ho
(Tonification)

Sha
(Sedation)

Some basic and common methods of treatment follow. Always try treating Kyo conditions first, then sedate the Jitsu symptoms. Often, tonifying only the Kyo condition can balance irregularities. It is very important to work only on the meridian which is in need of treatment. If the other meridians are fine, they should be left alone.

The common ways of applying Ho or Sha are detailed on the chart below. After diagnosis, first tonify the Kyo meridians. Generally, this action will sedate the Jitsu meridians. If not, you must apply Sha to sedate the Jitsu condition. Monitor the progress through continued diagnosis and treatment.

Condition	Kyo (depleted)	Jitsu (excess)
Treatment	Ho (tonify)	Sha (sedate)
Stroke the meridian	Stroke in the direction of the Ki flow	Stroke against the direction of the Ki flow
Massage before pressure to Tsubo?	Yes	No
Number and strength of applications of pressure to Tsubo	Using many light, repeated applications of pressure	Using a few, very strong applications of pressure
When to apply	While exhaling	While inhaling

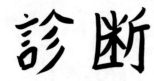

Shin Dan - Diagnosis

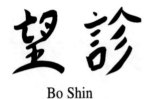

Bo Shin

Bun Shin

Mon Shin

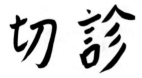

Setsu Shin

Diagnosis and Zoku Shin Do:

Zoku Shin Do developed from an ancient Chinese method of foot diagnosis and it is still used in traditional East Asian medicine as a general diagnostic method. It is used to assess irregular conditions in the internal organs through an examination of the feet. The practitioner follows foot diagnosis with other traditional Asian diagnostic methods to assess and treat specific irregularities.

Traditional East Asian medicine utilizes methods that differ from all other medicinal forms for determining physical conditions. These unique methods come from East Asian medical theory and are based on the Yin and Yang and the Five Elements theories. They have been used for at least 3,000 years, and possibly longer than 5,000 years. Mastering them requires time, practice, and patience. As you become more familiar with East Asian medicine, you will be able to diagnose specific conditions more accurately.

Traditionally, East Asian medical diagnosis is divided into four types. These are:

1) **Bo Shin** - diagnosis by first impression and observation of the client, without a close examination.
2) **Bun Shin** - diagnosis by listening to the character and quality of sounds a client makes. Note the tone or quality of the client's voice through shouting, laughing, singing, crying or groaning. Odors are also a component of this diagnosis.
3) **Mon Shin** - diagnosis by questioning. This consists of asking questions about the client's condition, either directly or by questionnaire. Inquire as to where the pain exists and what may have caused the condition. Questions should include health history and other health concerns.
4) **Setsu Shin** - diagnosis by examining the body. There are four basic methods of Setsu Shin which are briefly explained on the following page.

The best diagnoses combine the above methods. Use each method to discover possible causes and to eliminate other possibilities. Traditional East Asian medicine is individualized: it does not use Western medical pathological terminology. In Western medicine, two people may be diagnosed as having the same illness. This is rare in East Asian medicine because each individual's twelve internal organs will vary greatly in Kyo or Jitsu (see p. 26).

After performing Mon Shin, you should have some understanding of the client's condition. After asking a few questions, try to read the body as accurately as possible. Ask more questions to narrow the possible causes of the affliction. Then examine the body several times and communicate openly with the patient to make the best diagnosis possible.

Setsu Shin is a very fine and complex art. It is the actual examination of the body, the most important part of the diagnostic process. All methods of examinatio rely on the sensitivity in the therapist's fingertips. Keep in mind that just as Western medical doctors give different diagnoses and opinions based on the same set of information, Setsu Shin diagnoses will vary from therapist to therapist. The following are the main components of Setsu Shin:

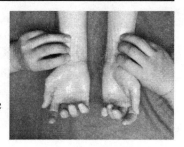

1) Myaku Shin - pulse diagnosis
2) Fuku Shin - hara (abdomen) diagnosis
3) Se Ko Shin - back diagnosis
4) Sek Kei - diagnosis by examining the meridians

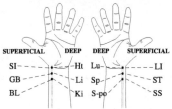

Myaku Shin - pulse diagnosis

Myaku Shin (pulse diagnosis) is the most important diagnosis in traditional East Asian medicine and it is considered one of most difficult procedures to master. It takes years of practice to recognize and understand all the information available in the pulse, but even beginners can usually recognize which meridians are normal or abnormal. Even a little information from a pulse diagnosis will assist your treatment.

Fuku Shin is used to diagnose the abdomen by noting slight differences in muscle tone and temperature. To evaluate the condition of the abdomen, consider five main measurements: 1) the stiffness of the muscle; 2) the sound it makes when gently tapped; 3) any temperature difference; 4) the amount of pain or discomfort from light pressure; and 5) the pulse from each corresponding location. By combining these five methods of diagnosis, you should be able to determine the condition of the internal organs. Each of the twelve internal organs has its own corresponding reflecting points, but these are not necessarily in the same area as the organ itself. One must learn the areas and what they represent. The picture at right is one of the most common charts showing the corresponding locations.

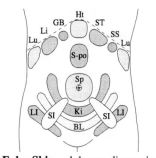

Fuku Shin - abdomen diagnosis

Se Ko Shin or Se Shin means examining the back to diagnose the condition of the body. It is the least used of the four methods of East Asian diagnosis. It is done by noting: 1) minor temperature differences; 2) tightness of muscles or muscular distortion; 3) pain, discomfort or over-sensitivity; and 4) pain and condition of the Yu Points. The Yu Points are located on both sides of the spine. They are important for both diagnosis and treatment. The diagram to the right shows the back regions and the corresponding parts of the individual meridians.

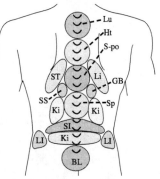

Se Ko Shin - back diagnosis

Sek Kei diagnosis is performed by lightly pinching the skin over the meridian lines to determine if there is any stagnation. If the client feels any pain, you have discovered exactly where stagnation is occurring on the meridian. Sek Kei is the easiest way to determine whether an irregularity is Kyo or Jitsu (Turn to p. 26 for explanations of Kyo and Jitsu).

Abbreviations			
Lung	Lu	Large Intestine	LI
Stomach	ST	Spleen	Sp
Heart	Ht	Small Intestine	SI
Bladder	BL	Kidney	Ki
Shin Po	S-po	San Sho	SS
Gall Bladder	GB	Liver	Li

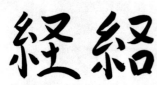

Keiraku -
Meridian System

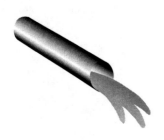

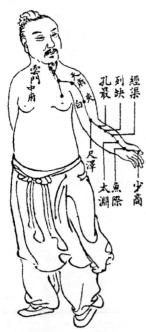

**Meridian illustration
from about 2600 B.C.**

Keiraku System:

Keiraku (commonly translated as "Meridian System") are the channels or pathways for Ki energy. Keiraku is traditionally used in Zoku Shin Do because it co-evolved with other forms of East Asian medicine such as Anma, acupuncture, moxibustion, and Kampo (Chinese herbology). Keiraku is a liquid vessel with a diameter of 20 to 55 millimicrons. It is the pathway for a transparent liquid (Toeki) that functions much like a nerve. Over the last two centuries the use of the Keiraku system with Japanese massage has become uncommon. One reason is that during that period of time Japanese massage had become primarily a job for the blind, and education was rarely supplied to them. The Keiraku system is not an easy system to master.

The Keiraku (Ching-Lo in Chinese) system consists of a total of 100 meridians and connections. The Keiraku is both a Kei system and a Raku system. The Kei system consists of thirty-two meridian vessels: twelve standard Kei meridians connected from internal organs, twelve branch meridians and eight vessels. The remainder is the Raku system and its connections.

The twelve standard Kei meridians are:

1)	Hai Kei	Lung Meridian
2)	Dai Cho Kei	Large Intestine Meridian
3)	I Kei	Stomach Meridian
4)	Hi Kei	Spleen Meridian
5)	Shin Kei	Heart Meridian
6)	Sho Cho Kei	Small Intestine Meridian
7)	Bo Ko Kei	Bladder Meridian
8)	Jin Kei	Kidney Meridian
9)	Shin Po Kei	Shin Po Meridian
10)	San Sho Kei	San Sho Meridian
11)	Tan Kei	Gall Bladder Meridian
12)	Kan Kei	Liver Meridian

The twelve Kei meridians are connected to each other in the order listed above to form a giant loop. Because the meridians are found on both sides of the body (they are bilaterally symmetrical), there are two loops, one on each side of the body. It takes exactly twenty-four hours for Ki to cycle through the twelve meridians.

The eight vessels divide the body in different directions to balance the meridians. The two vessels which travel along the median line on the front and the back are the two most often used for treatment.

13)	Nin Myaku	- Conception vessel
14)	Toku Myaku	- Governing vessel

These two vessels are combined with the twelve standard Kei meridians to become what is commonly called the "fourteen meridians on the body". These are most commonly used for diagnosis and treatment in East Asian medicine.

Tsubo:

When we feel aches or pains, it is a natural response to touch the painful area in order to find the exact source of pain. Simply rubbing or applying pressure to these points often eases the pain. The conceptualization of tsubo originated in China over 3,000 years ago, in response to the discovery that certain painful points located on the body were common in all people. Since that time, tsubo has become a well developed system. This concept forms the foundation of massage, traditional Chinese medicine, and Zoku Shin Do.

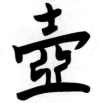

Tsubo - Acupoints

Tsubo is often translated in English as "acupoint" or "acupuncture point". In my teaching and in this book, however, I refer to these as tsubo. Tsubo can be stimulated to relieve pain, to produce certain effects in the internal organs, and/or to relieve symptoms. Using tsubo and Keiraku when applying Japanese foot massage can be a very effective form of treatment.

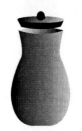

The character for tsubo originated in China at least 3,000 years ago. It is a Chinese hieroglyph that literally means "jar". On the body, a tsubo is shaped something like a jar or pore (see right). It is helpful to visualize a meridian as a hose with water running through it. The liquid (Toeki) carries bioelectricity (Ki) throughout the body. A tsubo is a point where stagnation commonly occurs on the meridian, just as kinks in a hose will prevent the water from flowing freely.

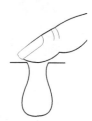

There are two categories of tsubo: Kei Ketsu and Ki Ketsu. Kei Ketsu tsubo exist on top of the twelve meridians and two vessels. There are about 361 of these on each side of the body (see chart for the number of tsubo on each meridian). Ki Ketsu tsubo are not on the meridians. There are about 750 of these on each side of the body. The study of tsubo focuses mainly on Kei Ketsu. These can be thought of as a stagnation point or counterpoint on the meridian.

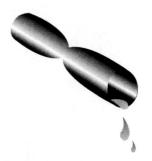

Stimulating the precise location of tsubo is essential for treatment. If the practitioner is off by even 1/16 of an inch, effective treatment is not possible. Tsubo are generally located near the tip of a nerve or at a physical "weak spot", such as between the muscles and bones. You will usually find tsubo in slight depressions or indentations on the body. Through physical examination, these depressions can help you to locate the exact spot of the tsubo. The best way to learn the location of tsubo is to try to identify tsubo on your own body. This way, you can feel the different sensations of pain and pressure at each point, while learning the precise location of tsubo on the body.

Pain on a particular tsubo is often an indication of some irregularity in the physical body and/or internal organs. But some tsubo may reflect a variety of conditions, so if two people have similar pain in a particular tsubo, it does not mean that their conditions are identical.

Listed below are the number of Tsubo in each meridian:

Lung	11
Large Intestine	20
Stomach	45
Spleen	21
Heart	9
Small Intestine	19
Bladder	67
Kidney	27
Shin Po	9
San Sho	23
Gall Bladder	44
Liver	14
Nin Myaku	24
Toku Myaku	28

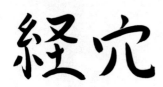

Kei Ketsu -
Tsubo on meridians

The Meridians and the Tsubo of the Feet

Tsubo is the most important concept for effective application of Zoku Shin Do. Proper application of pressure to the appropriate tsubo ensures the release of stagnating Ki. Throughout this book each treatment is based upon locating the proper tsubo and applying the appropriate pressure to that point (see p. 94 for further instructions on this topic).

Out of 361 tsubo points, most acupuncturists and East Asian body-workers commonly use from 130 to 200 tsubo during a treatment. The other points are used for less common circumstances, and it is rare that a practitioner uses all of the tsubo points. Certain tsubo points are used to treat an array of illnesses, while other points are used for conditions so rare that a therapist may never find the opportunity to use them.

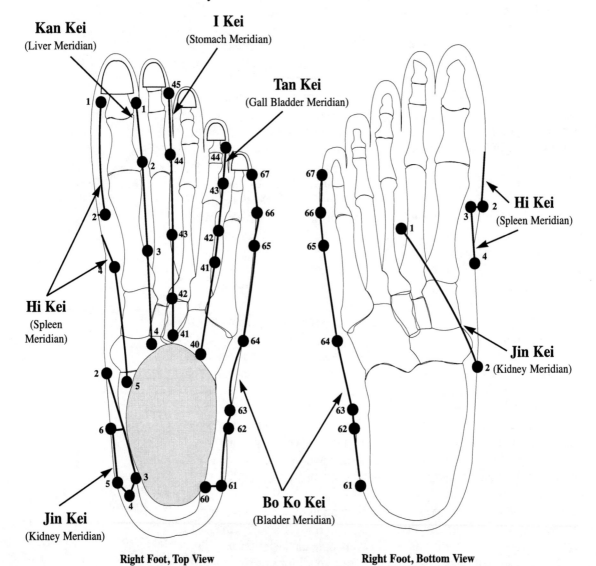

Right Foot, Top View

Right Foot, Bottom View

The Meridians and the Tsubo of the Legs

There are six meridians running on the legs, three Yin meridians and three Yang meridians.

The three Yin meridians are the Kidney Meridian (Jin Kei), the Spleen Meridian (Hi Kei), and the Liver Meridian (Kan Kei). Jin Kei begins on the bottom of the foot, while Hi Kei and Kan Kei begin at the corners of the big toe. All three run along the inside of the legs, up into the front part of the torso and end in the chest.

The three Yang meridians are the Gall Bladder Meridian (Tan Kei), the Stomach Meridian (I Kei), and the Bladder Meridian (Bo Ko Kei). These all begin near the eyes.

I Kei stays in the front of the body and legs, Tan Kei runs along the side of the body and legs, and Bo Ko Kei runs down the back next to the spine, then through the back of the legs. All three Yang meridians finish on the tops of the toes at the corner of a toenail.

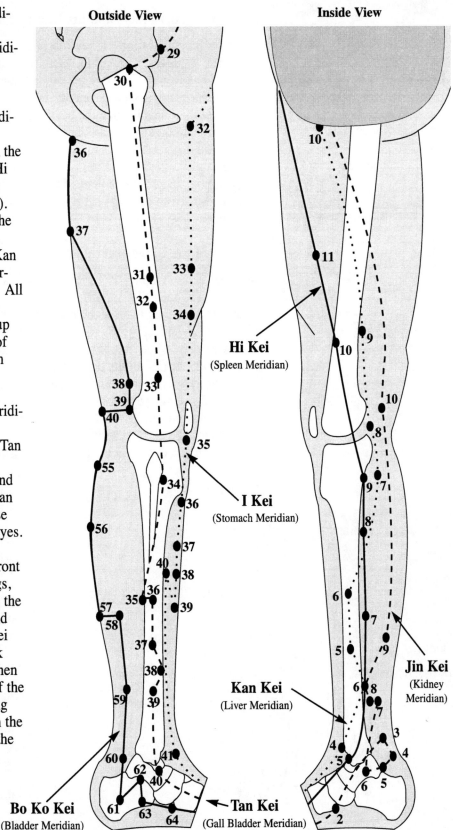

Outside View

Inside View

Hi Kei
(Spleen Meridian)

I Kei
(Stomach Meridian)

Kan Kei
(Liver Meridian)

Jin Kei
(Kidney Meridian)

Bo Ko Kei
(Bladder Meridian)

Tan Kei
(Gall Bladder Meridian)

腎経

Jin Kei - Kidney Meridian

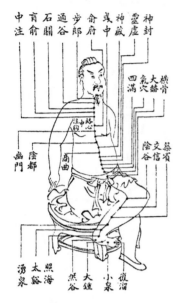

中育石通步俞炁神靈神
注俞關谷郎府中藏虚封

四氣大横
满穴赫骨

注中神心
個府

陰交築
谷信賓

幽陰都
門曲

湧太照
泉谿海

然大小復
谷鐘泉溜

Jin Kei - Kidney Meridian

Function of the Kidneys and the Kidney Meridian

The main function of the Kidney Meridian is to support the kidneys. The kidneys govern all the activities which concern liquid and fluid levels in the body. The body's liquids include light, clear, surfice fluids such as sweat, tears, saliva, and skin moisture, while the fluids include the heavier, yellow, inner fluid that protect internal organs. The kidneys are also responsible for the storage and distribution of Shin (essences, somewhat similar to hormones in Western medicine), which govern birth, growth, reproduction, and developement. The kidneys are responsible for bones and marrow, ears and hearing, hair and hair follicles, and will power.

Pathway of the Kidney Meridian

The first point on the Kidney Meridian is in the center of the sole of the foot (Kidney #1, Yu Sen). From there, the meridian travels toward the upper edge of the heel pad at the base of the arch, (Kidney #2, Nen Koku). Next, it travels up behind and below the ankle bones where it loops (the only meridian to do so), and travels up the ankle. It juts forward to meet the Spleen and Liver Meridians (Spleen #6, San In Ko), and then follows the posterior and medial side of the calf. From there, it runs past the knee, along the medial side of the thigh, and up the front of the abdomen to the chest. Here it stays one inch out from the medial line of the body, ending at the base of the clavicle (Kidney #27, Yu Fu).

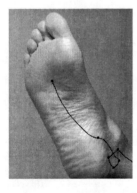

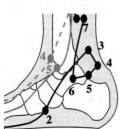

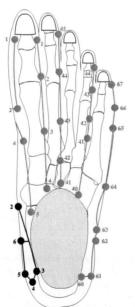

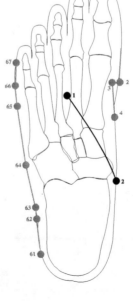

Kidney #1 Yu Sen
- Kidney problems
- High blood pressure

Kidney #2 Nen Koku
- Pain on sole of the foot
- High blood pressure

Kidney #3 Tai Kei
- Abnormal constipation
- impotence

Kidney #4 Tai Sho
- Inability to urinate
- Pain on heel of the foot

Kidney #5 Sui Sen
- Pain on heel of the foot
- Pain in the ankle

Kidney #6 Sho Kai
- Menstral tensions
- Insomnia

Hi Kei - Spleen Meridian

Function of the Spleen and the Spleen Meridian

The main function of the Spleen Meridian is to support the spleen. For women, the Spleen Meridian regulates menstruation. The spleen controls the ketsu (similar to blood in Western medicine), by removing the damaged or destroyed blood cells from the bloodstream. It is responsible for general filtering in the body. It also regulates the amount of Ki that both the stomach and small intestines supply to the heart.

Pathway of the Spleen Meridian

The Spleen Meridian begins at the inside corner of the big toe nail and runs along the side of the foot through the top of the arch. From here, it continues up the inside of the lower leg until it crosses to the front of the leg just above the knee. It then follows the outside of the abdomen until it turns outward just one inch below Lung #1 (Chu Fu). It ends six inches below the center of the axilla (underarm), halfway between the axilla and the eleventh rib.

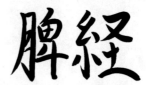

Hi Kei - Spleen Meridian

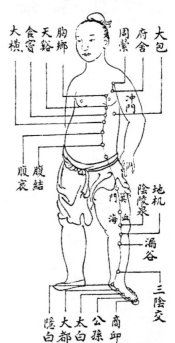

Spleen #1 In Paku
- Diarrhea
- Excessive menstruation

Spleen #2 Tai To
- Abdominal pain
- Vomiting

Spleen #3 Tai Haku
- Arthritis in the big toe
- Diarrhea

Spleen #4 Ko Son
- Menstrual pain
- Heart pain

Spleen #5 Sho Kyu
- Hemorrhoids
- Pain in the ankle

Spleen #6 San In Ko
(avoid during 1st trimester of pregnancy)
- Menstrual irregularity and pain
- High blood pressure

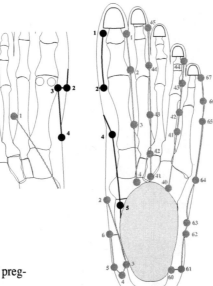

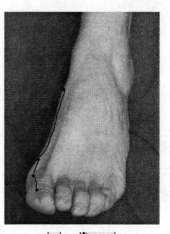

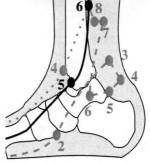

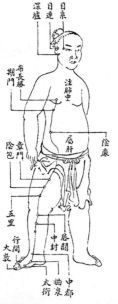

肝経

Kan Kei - Liver Meridian

Kan Kei - Liver Meridian

Function of the Liver and the Liver Meridian

The Liver Meridian supports the liver in performing its functions. The liver is responsible for controlling the quality and quantity of the blood. The main function of the liver is to purify and store the blood. It does not have anything to do with blood pressure in the body; it only controls the total amount of blood circulating through the body. The liver also creates immune cells and digestive enzymes, as well as resistance to outside infections or invasions.

Pathway of the Liver Meridian

The Liver Meridian begins at the lateral tip of the big toe at the corner of the nail bed and flows into the foot, staying on the lateral edge of the first metatarsal. At the base of the ankle, it runs up the front and inside part of the ankle and juts in to meet the Kidney and Spleen Meridians (Spleen #6, San In Ko). It then continues up along the front inside corner of the leg, around the inside of the knee where the Spleen Meridian crosses it, and up the inside of the leg.

From here, the Liver Meridian enters into the abdomen and stays between the Spleen and Stomach meridians until it is even with the navel. From this point, the Liver Meridian runs out to the tip of the eleventh rib (Liver #13, Sho Mon), and then follows the rib cage back inside to finish about midway between the xyphoid process and the side of the body at the base of the rib cage (Liver #14, Ki Mon).

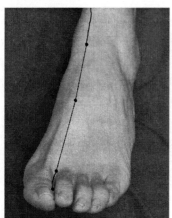

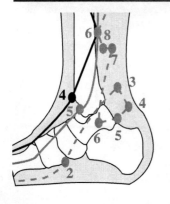

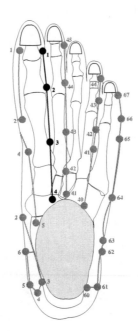

Liver #1 Dai Ton
- Urinary disorders
- Constipation

Liver #2 Ko Kan
- Vomiting
- Abdominal cramps

Liver #3 Tai Sho
(avoid during pregnancy)
- Abdominal cramps
- Gout

Liver #4 Chu Ho
- Irregular menstruation
- Dysmenorrhea

I Kei - Stomach Meridian

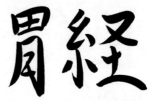

Function of the Stomach and the Stomach Meridian

The main function of the Stomach Meridian is to support the functioning of the Spleen Meridian. It also aids the stomach. The primary function of the stomach is to begin breaking down food with acid and send the remnants to the small intestines. After chewing, it executes the second stage of breaking down of food so that it can be further digested in the intestines. The stomach is also responsible for sending Ki to the heart.

I Kei - Stomach Meridian

Pathway of the Stomach Meridian

The Stomach Meridian begins just below the middle of the eye and travels straight down the cheek bone to the outside corner of the lips before turning towards the middle of the cheekbone where it splits (Stomach #5). From here, one fork follows the jawbone, runs up to the front of the ear, ending at the top corner of the forehead (Stomach #8). The other fork moves down from the jawbone and along the front of the the throat to the top of the clavicle. From there, it moves laterally along the top of the clavicle to the middle of the clavicle, then down the chest and abdomen between the Liver and Kidney Meridians. At the base of the trunk, it runs laterally to the front of the leg and then down. It runs just lateral to the kneecap and slightly lateral to the tibia. Midway down, it temporarily angles laterally, before continuing back down the front of the leg and ankle. It ends between the second and third metatarsals and the corner of the nail of the second toe.

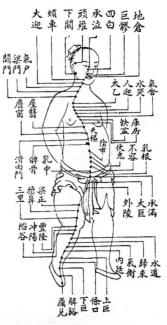

Stomach #41 Kai Kei
- Constipation
- Pain in the ankle

Stomach #42 Sho Yo
- Loss of appetite
- Vomiting

Stomach #43 Kan Koku
- Gastrointestinal pain
- Pain on dorsal side of the foot

Stomach #44 Nai Tei
- Diarrhea
- Sore throat

Stomach #45 Rei Da
- Upset stomach
- Insomnia

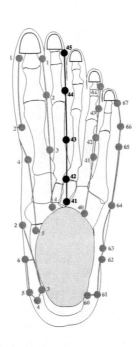

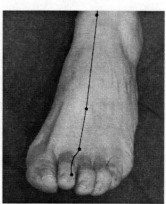

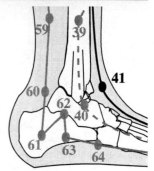

胆経

**Tan Kei -
Gall Bladder Meridian**

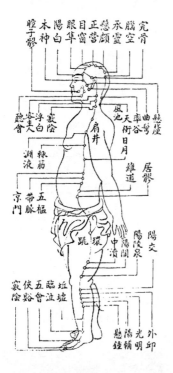

Tan Kei - Gall Bladder Meridian

Function of the Gall Bladder and the Gall Bladder Meridian

The main function of the Gall Bladder Meridian is to support the functioning of the Gall Bladder. The main function of the Gall Bladder in East Asian medicine is to support the Liver. Usually the Gall Bladder is responsible for breaking down the fatty foods in our diets by storing and distributing bile.

Pathway of the Gall Bladder Meridian

The Gall Bladder Meridian begins at the lateral corner of the eye, travels to the front of the ear at the upper corner of the hair line, and then to back behind the ear. From here, it runs to the middle of the forehead (Gall Bladder #14), back over the head and down to the base of the skull (Gall Bladder #20), just lateral to the Bladder Meridian. Next it travels to the top of the suprascapular region, forward over the scapula, and along the inside edge of the anterior deltoid. From here, the Gall Bladder Meridian follows the side of the body, with a detour near the end of the Liver Meridian, then back across the side of the body to the Kidney Bo Point at the base of the 12th rib (Gall Bladder #25). Next, it curves down to the top of the pelvis bone, moves slightly into the buttocks, and follows the lower edge of the gluteus maximus to the side of the leg. The Gall Bladder Meridian follows the lateral side of the leg down to the top of the ankle, and runs just above the ankle bone. It finishes by traveling down the dorsal side of the foot, between the fourth and fifth metatarsals, and ends on the lateral corner of the fourth toe.

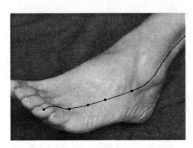

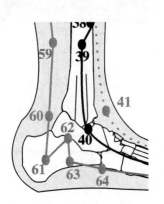

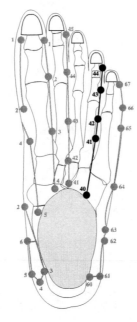

Gall Bladder #40 Kyu Kyo
- Lumbar pain
- Pain in the calf muscle

Gall Bladder #41 (Ashi no) Rin Kyu
- Irregular menstruation
- Arthritis

Gall Bladder #42 Chi Go E
- Tinnitus
- Chest pain

Gall Bladder #43 Kyo Kei
- Hearing loss
- Dizziness

Gall Bladder #44 (Ashi no) Kyo In
- Inflammation in the throat
- Asthma

Bo Ko Kei - Bladder Meridian

Function of the Bladder and the Bladder Meridian

The main function of the Bladder Meridian is to support the kidneys and the Kidney Meridian. The Bladder Meridian is also responsible for the functioning of the bladder, which eliminates waste water from the body. Its function is similar to that of the Kidney Meridian, but it is also responsible for the overall balance of all of the internal organs.

Pathway of the Bladder Meridian

The Bladder Meridian begins at the inside corner of the eye and runs straight up over the forehead and scalp, and down the back of the head to the base of the skull (Bladder #10) where it splits. One fork (Inner Bladder Meridian) runs next to the vertebrae to the sacrum, along the base of the buttocks, and down the back of the leg. The other fork (Outer Bladder Meridian) runs parallel and slightly lateral to the first fork, on the other side of the erector muscles as it travels down the back. It then runs down the back of the buttocks and down the back of the leg, again, slightly lateral to the Inner Bladder Meridian. The two reunite just above the back of the knee. The Bladder Meridian then travels down the back of the leg, and follows laterally along the achilles' tendon. Finally, it goes under the ankle bone, and along the dorsal and lateral edge of the foot to the fifth (pinky) toe, where it ends on the lateral corner of the nail.

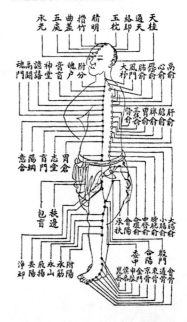

膀胱経

**Bo Ko Kei -
Bladder Meridian**

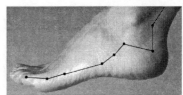

Bladder #60 Kon Ron
- Headache
- Lumbar pain

Bladder #61 Boku Shin
- Weakness in the leg
- Pain on heel of the foot

Bladder #62 Shin Myaku
- Menstrual pain
- Headache

Bladder #63 Kin Mon
(acupuncture treatment only)
- paralysis

Bladder #64 Kei Kotsu
- Lumbar pain
- Urination problems

Bladder #65 Soku Kotsu
- Diarrhea
- Lumbar pain

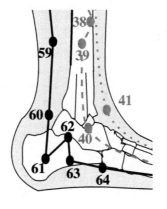

Bladder #66 Tsuu Koku
- Dizziness
- Headache

Bladder #67 Shin In
(avoid during pregnancy)
- Headache
- General body pain

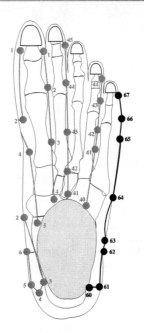

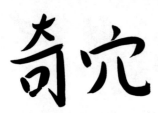

Ki Ketsu
- Extraordinary Point

Ki Ketsu - Extraordinary Point

Ki Ketsu literally translates as "strange hole", but is more commonly known as "extraordinary point" or "strange point". As I have briefly explained on page 27, Ki Ketsu refers to a tsubo on the body that does not belong to any meridian. There are more than 650 Ki Ketsu points, twice as many as Kei Ketsu (tsubo on the meridians). Ki Ketsu may be on the meridian line, but this does not necessarily mean that it belongs to that meridian. Ki Ketsu points do not directly relate to meridian balance, but are normally manipulated to treat specific conditions.

Here are a few of the well-known Ki Ketsu points on the feet and their functions.

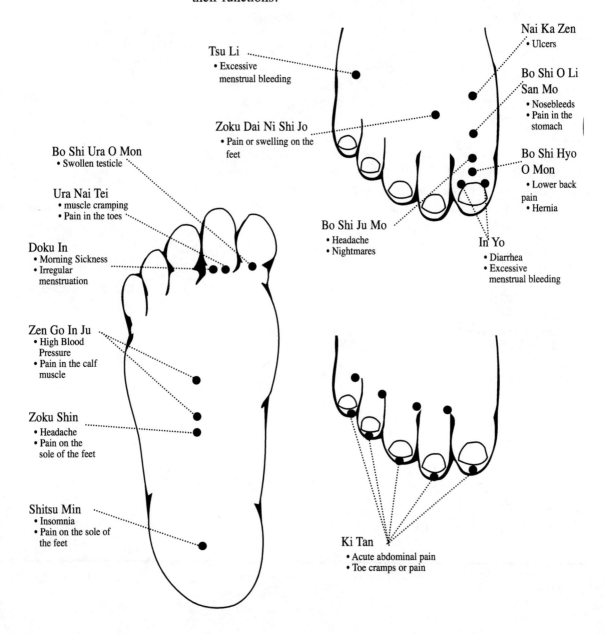

Tsu Li
• Excessive menstrual bleeding

Zoku Dai Ni Shi Jo
• Pain or swelling on the feet

Nai Ka Zen
• Ulcers

Bo Shi O Li San Mo
• Nosebleeds
• Pain in the stomach

Bo Shi Hyo O Mon
• Lower back pain
• Hernia

Bo Shi Ju Mo
• Headache
• Nightmares

In Yo
• Diarrhea
• Excessive menstrual bleeding

Bo Shi Ura O Mon
• Swollen testicle

Ura Nai Tei
• muscle cramping
• Pain in the toes

Doku In
• Morning Sickness
• Irregular menstruation

Zen Go In Ju
• High Blood Pressure
• Pain in the calf muscle

Zoku Shin
• Headache
• Pain on the sole of the feet

Shitsu Min
• Insomnia
• Pain on the sole of the feet

Ki Tan
• Acute abdominal pain
• Toe cramps or pain

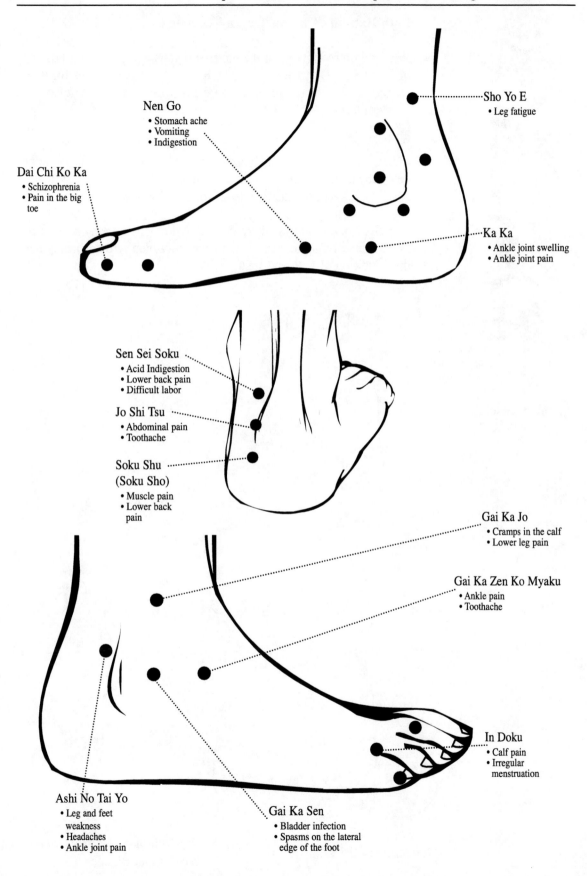

Nen Go
- Stomach ache
- Vomiting
- Indigestion

Sho Yo E
- Leg fatigue

Dai Chi Ko Ka
- Schizophrenia
- Pain in the big toe

Ka Ka
- Ankle joint swelling
- Ankle joint pain

Sen Sei Soku
- Acid Indigestion
- Lower back pain
- Difficult labor

Jo Shi Tsu
- Abdominal pain
- Toothache

Soku Shu (Soku Sho)
- Muscle pain
- Lower back pain

Gai Ka Jo
- Cramps in the calf
- Lower leg pain

Gai Ka Zen Ko Myaku
- Ankle pain
- Toothache

In Doku
- Calf pain
- Irregular menstruation

Ashi No Tai Yo
- Leg and feet weakness
- Headaches
- Ankle joint pain

Gai Ka Sen
- Bladder infection
- Spasms on the lateral edge of the foot

臓腑反射

Zofu Hansha

Zofu Hansha - Internal Organ Reflection

Working on reflections of the internal organs is a very important part of Zoku Shin Do treatment. Note that the East Asian terms for the physiological functioning of the internal organs are different from the Western terms.

Particular internal organs and regions of the body reflect to specific regions of the feet. Zofu Hansha is the first and oldest method to be developed, and has been using these regions to diagnosis and treat conditions and ailments by way of the feet for over 5000 years.

The chart below shows where the internal organs reflect on the feet. For treatment, application must be carefully modified according to the condition of Kyo and Jitsu.

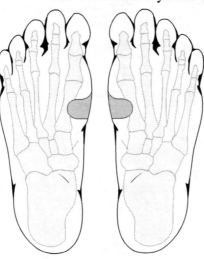

Reflection of the Stomach

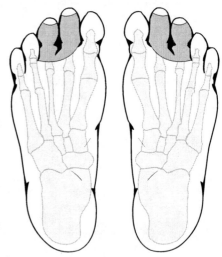

Reflection of the Eyes

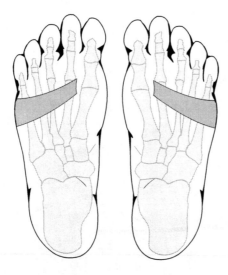

Reflection of the Lungs

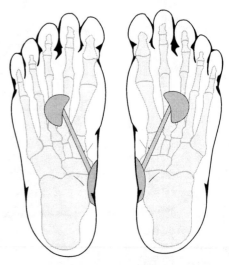

Reflection of the Kidney, Ureter and Bladder

Keiraku Hansha - Meridian Reflections

Another unique property of Zoku Shin Do is that it also works with the reflections of the meridians. Six of the actual meridians run into the feet, so you can work directly on these meridians through the feet. The meridians in the arms do not run to the foot. The only way you can treat arm meridians such as the lung, heart, or large intestines, is to use the reflections of the meridians.

When you work on the reflections of the meridians, it is necessary for you to work very gently on a surface level. You can combine working on the reflections of meridians with working on the actual meridians, by stroking them both to enhance the effectiveness of a treatment.

In Asia, some Zoku Shin Do practitioners use the reflection of the meridians extensively, while some practitioners do not use them at all. Meridian reflection is a very effective tool in maximizing the effect of the overall Zoku Shin Do treatment.

The chart below shows two examples of the reflection of meridians.

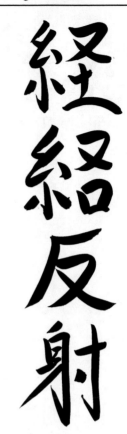

Keiraku Hansha

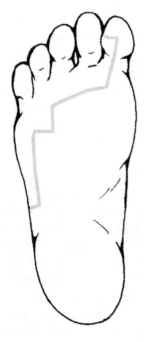

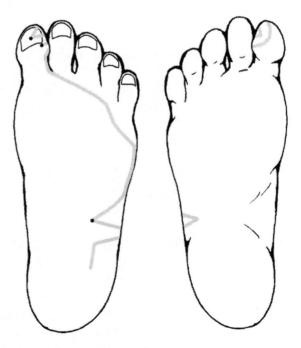

Reflection of the
Small Intestines Meridian

Reflection of the
Gall Bladder Meridian

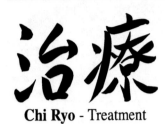

Chi Ryo - Treatment

Procedures of Zoku Shin Do Treatment

Treating specific conditions with Zoku Shin Do is unique because East Asian medicine has a different understanding of pathology than Western medicine. Zoku Shin Do also has very different methods of diagnosis. In this section, I will show three clinical examples of common ailments which highlight the treatment properties of Zoku Shin Do.

As I have explained previously, Zoku Shin Do combines five major methods of treatment (see p. 21). During treatment, it is uncommon to use all five methods. Combining 2 - 3 of the methods for application will usually ensure the effectiveness of Zoku Shin Do treatment. Zoku Shin Do does not have a fixed treatment procedure, such as having a specific point to press or a specific meridian to work on, relative to the symptoms of a condition. From the view of East Asian medicine, the condition of health for each individual is different, and two people may have similar sypmtoms, it is difficult to find two people with exactly same the condition (see Diagnosis, pp. 28-29).

Unlike other methods of reflexology, Zoku Shin Do treats only according to individual diagnosis. For example, if two people suffer from insomnia, it does not mean that you will treat one with the same procedure as you treat the other. One person may suffer from insomnia caused by the digestive system, while the other may suffer from insomnia caused by a condition of the liver. You must treat each person differently according to individual diagnoses.

Even a single client coming in at a different time with the same symptoms as a previous time might be treated differently, according to the diagnosis. This means that the conditions for each treatment change and you must adjust the treatment to cater to those conditions in order to provide the most effective treatment. Since Asian pathological terminology is so different from Western terminology, this will require good understanding of East Asian medical theory.

As you become more familiar with Zoku Shin Do treatment, you will increase your sense for which method of treatment will work for which set of circumstances. Dependent upon the conditions, certain methods are known to work superior to others, but of course this will fluctuate from client to client. For example, you could find yourself treating insomnia, which generally concerns the digestive system. If you detect irregularity in the stomach, small intestines, and large intestinal meridians or organs, you will apply treatment to those organs or meridians. If the condition is Kyo (depleted), you must Ho (tonify). If the condition is Jitsu (excessive), you must Sha (sedate). The same condition could also be treated through the tsubo, like the extraordinary point Shitsu Min (see p 40). Some points are known to be very effective when treating specific conditions of health.

Zoku Shin Do can help muscular skeletal problems as well, such as sore neck, stiff shoulders, or back ache. These conditions can also use muscular skeletal reflections, as well as meridian reflections, for effective treatment.

Another advantage of Zoku Shin Do, is that it is excellent for treating emotional imbalances, through the Five Elements method. Various psychological and emotional conditions are reflections of internal organ imbalances, and you can restore imbalanced emotions by balancing the internal organs and meridians. For example, irregularities in the lung commonly cause sadness or depression. Often, the lung and lung meridians are worked on to treat excessive sadness and depression.

Chapter Four

ANATOMY OF THE FEET

Performing Japanese foot massage does not require knowledge or experience of other styles of massage, nor is it necessary to have a complete understanding of the anatomy or physiology of the feet to give a good foot massage. Of course, this information is helpful and will be briefly introduced as necessary. In the East, we have been giving foot massage for over 5000 years, yet have only understood the anatomy and physiology of the human body for less than 200 years. In massage therapy, it is more important to understand anatomy with one's hands, than to possess a complete academic knowledge of it. The study of technical anatomy is helpful, however, and you may find that it compliments your massage practice.

Anatomy language is used to communicate between therapists to minimize confusion. For example, the top of the foot can be understood as being around the toes, or for some people, as the dorsal of the foot. Some people consider the inside and outside of the foot to be the toes and the heel. This chapter explains basic terminology to help reduce misunderstanding during explanations of the techniques. This book (the popular edition) has eliminated most of the anatomical terminology and has substituted simpler phrases, keeping necessary terminiology in parenthesis.

The pictures and diagrams in this chapter show the basic structure of the bones, muscles and ligaments in the feet. The only information which will be critical for you to know to use this book are the locations of the first through fifth metatarsals and the phalanges (toes). These should be very easy to memorize, however, and should not take much time to learn. Although the exact skeletal and muscular structures of each foot are different, these diagrams provide general guidelines to work from.

Inner Hand and Outer Hand

In this book, you will occasionally see the terms "inner hand" and "outer hand". The inner hand is the hand which is nearest to the center of the client's body. For example, if you are seated at the client's feet and working on the client's right foot, your right hand is considered to be the inner hand.

The outer hand is the hand closest to the outer edge of the client's body or closest to the smallest toe. Your left hand would be considered your outer hand, using the same example from the previous paragraph.

I use the term "inner thumb" or "inner fingers" and "outer thumb" or "outer fingers". This refers to the thumb or fingers of the inner hand or the thumb or fingers of the outer hand.

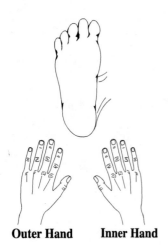

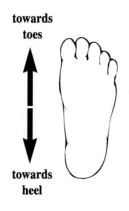

Outer Hand   **Inner Hand**

towards toes

towards heel

For the sake of consistency, all of the examples shown in this book are demonstrated and explained on the client's right foot. I have arranged the text this way because most people find it easier to learn on the right foot. To work on the left foot, follow the directions with reversed hand positions. Each example should be performed on both feet. Be sure to practice on the right and left foot until you are comfortable with both. In an actual foot massage, it is common to completely work on one foot before working on the other.

Plantar, Dorsal, Medial and Lateral

Plantar is the underside or sole of the foot. Dorsal is the top of the foot. Medial refers to the center line in between the feet (by the arch or big toe) or a motion in that direction. Lateral refers to the outside edges of the feet or a motion in that direction. We will use these terms to minimize confusion. For example, the "top (dorsal) of the foot" would mean the top side or dorsal side of the foot, not necessarily on the toes.

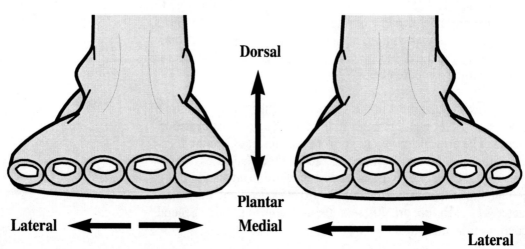

Dorsal

Plantar

Lateral ⟵ ⟶ **Medial**   **Lateral** ⟵ ⟶

Specific Regions of the Feet

These are brief definitions of terms used to describe different regions of the feet. Each example describes a slightly different area of the feet.

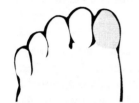 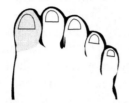

Big Toe (Great Toe or Large Toe)
The entire first phalange of the foot - from where it joins the foot to its tip.

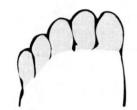 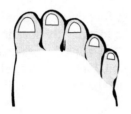

Toes
All of the phalanges from where they connect to the foot to the tips. On occasion, the Big Toe is classified separately. When this is the case,"Toes" refers to the other phalanges.

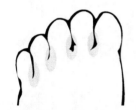 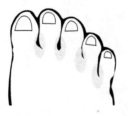

Webbing
The fleshy areas between the toes and foot. Webbing is found on both the plantar and dorsal sides of the foot.

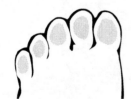 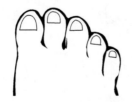

Balls of the Toes
The ends of the distal phalanges and the pads surrounding them on the plantar side of each toe. In a regular standing position, the balls of the toes will be the only parts of the toes touching the ground.

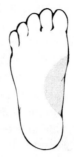

Arch
The medial region of the foot between the edge of the heel pad and the ball of the foot. (medial longitudinal arch)

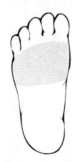

Balls of the Feet
The joint regions of the metatarsals and the phalanges on the plantar side of the foot.

Heel
The region around the heel including the heel pad as well as the heel bone.

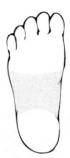

Middle of the Foot
The plantar side of the foot between the ball of the foot and the heel pad. This is where the metatarsals are found.

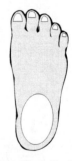

Top (Dorsal) of the Foot
The entire upper surface of the foot from the ankle to the toe nails.

Edges of the Heel
The outside rims of the heel pads surrounding, but not including, the heel bone.

Bones of the Feet

The foot has a relatively complex bone structure which is similar to the hand, the biggest difference being that the arm is connected to the end of the hand, while the leg is connected to the top of the foot. This means that the leg sits on the top of the talus bone and not the end of the calcaneus bone. The complex skeletal system of the foot allows it to move in many different directions. This helps to support different complex functions such as inward and outward rotation (inversion and eversion), movement of the toes (extension and flexion), and many other movements that generally combine together to create simple functions of the ankle and foot. The foot is constructed with three different directions of arches, which allows it the ability to support and balance the entire bodyweight during the complex functioning of the human body.

When studying Japanese foot massage, familiarizing yourself with how the bones run in the foot and the location of metatarsals and phalanges can be helpful. The phalanges and metatarsals are counted from the medial side of the foot to the lateral side. For example, the bones of the big toe would be the first metatarsal and first phalange.

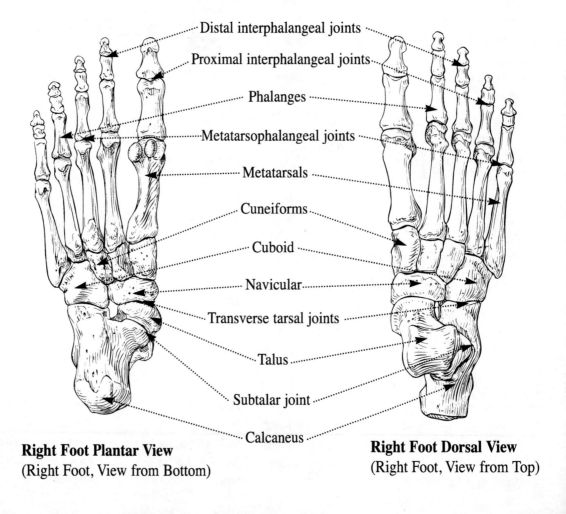

Distal interphalangeal joints

Proximal interphalangeal joints

Phalanges

Metatarsophalangeal joints

Metatarsals

Cuneiforms

Cuboid

Navicular

Transverse tarsal joints

Talus

Subtalar joint

Calcaneus

Right Foot Plantar View
(Right Foot, View from Bottom)

Right Foot Dorsal View
(Right Foot, View from Top)

Right Foot Medial View
(Right Foot, View from Inside Edge)

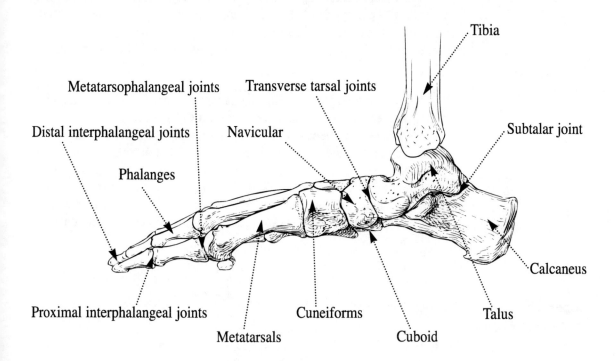

Right Foot Lateral View
(Right Foot, View from Outside Edge)

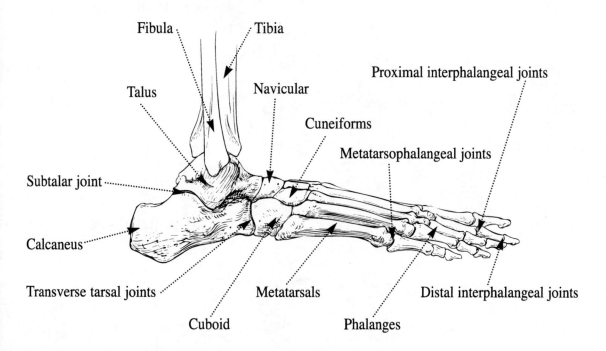

Muscles and Tendons of the Feet

The muscles and tendons of the feet are very complex. It takes many muscles performing specialized functions to support all of the activities of the feet, and they are commonly divided into three separate layers. Some of the foot muscles are connected to the lower legs to produce ankle and foot movements.

It is not critical to memorize the name for every single muscle and tendon of the foot. It is more important to have some idea of where the muscles and tendons are located, how big they are, and in which direction they are running. The majority of the muscles run from the heel to the toe, but there are a few muscles that run the transverse direction across the metatarsals. The major muscles and tendons are shown here, but for a more detailed understanding of the anatomy of the foot, it is best to refer to a good anatomy or cadaver reference book.

Superficial Layer of Planter Muscles:
Right Foot Plantar View
(Right Foot, View from Bottom)

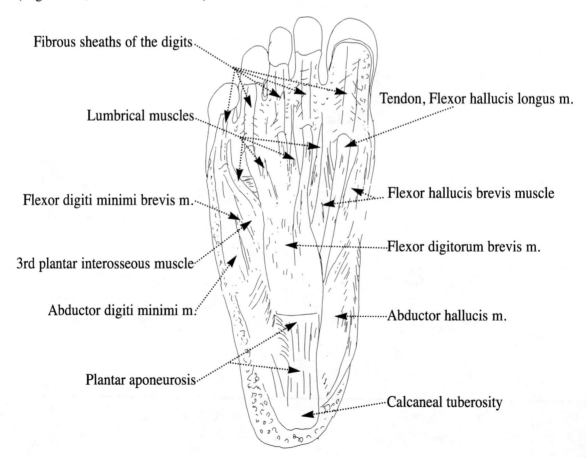

Fibrous sheaths of the digits

Lumbrical muscles

Tendon, Flexor hallucis longus m.

Flexor digiti minimi brevis m.

Flexor hallucis brevis muscle

3rd plantar interosseous muscle

Flexor digitorum brevis m.

Abductor digiti minimi m.

Abductor hallucis m.

Plantar aponeurosis

Calcaneal tuberosity

**Middle Layer of Planter Muscles:
Right Foot Plantar View**
(Right Foot, View from Bottom)

Tendons, Flexor digitorum brevis m.

Abductor hallucis m.
(transverse head)

Lumbrical mm.

Flexor digiti minimi m.

Abductor digiti minimi m.

Plantar interosseous muscles

Peroneus longus muscle

Quadratus plantae m.

Abductor digiti minimi muscle

Tendons, Flexor hallus longus m.

Tendons, Flexor
digitorum long. m.

Flexor Hallucis longus m.

Tendon, Flexor dig-
itorum longus m.

Tendons, Flexor
hallucis longus m.

Abductor hallucis m.

Abductor digiti minimi
muscle (deep head)

Flexor digitorum brevis m.

Calcaneal tuberosity

**Deep Layer of Planter Muscles:
Right Foot Plantar View**
(Right Foot, View from Bottom)

Tendons, Flexor dig-
itorum longus m.

Tendons of lumbrical mm.

Plantar interosseus muscle

Opponens digiti minimi m.

Flexor digiti minimi m.

Abductor digiti
minimi m.

Tendon, Peroneus
longus muscle

Quadratus plantae m.

Long plantar ligament

Tendons, Flexor
digitorum longus m.

Abductor digiti minimi m.

Flexor digitorum brevis m.

Tendons, Flexor
hallucis longus m.

Tendons, Flexor
digitorum brevis m.

Abductor hallucis
(transverse head)

Abductor hallucis
(oblique head)

Flexor hallucis brevis m.

Abductor hallucis m.

Tendon, Flexor
hallucis longus m.

Tendon, Flexor
digit. longus m.

Tendon, Tibialis
posterior m.

Flexor retinaculum

Abductor hallucis m.

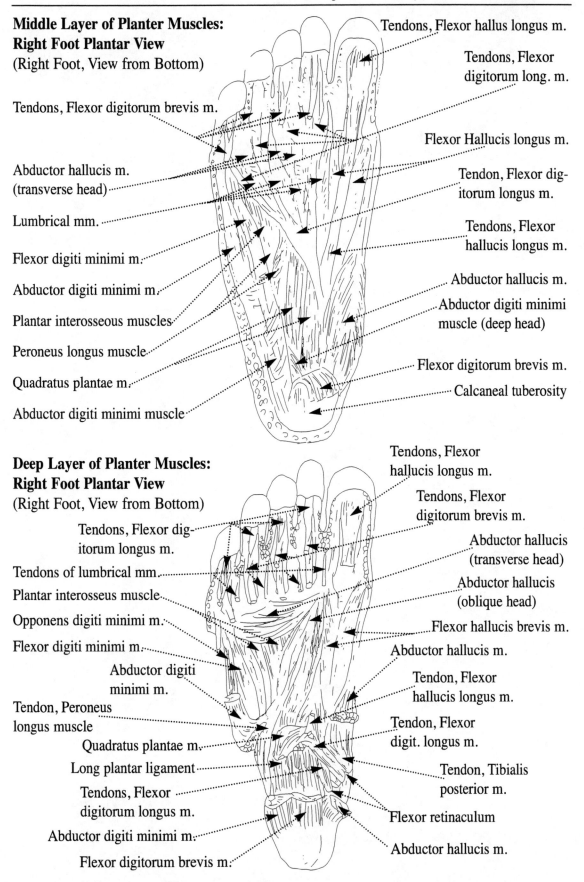

Chapter Five

THE APPLICATION OF
JAPANESE FOOT MASSAGE

In this chapter, I will explain the basics for application of Japanese foot massage, precautions, and provide basic information to help you better perform Japanese foot massage, such as how to set up a table or work on the floor. I will also provide ideas for protection and maintenance of your hands during application which you may find useful with any modality of massage and bodywork. This chapter should answer the most common questions about the application of Japanese foot massage.

Whether you already are proficient in other massage forms, or a raw beginner, you should practice massage on a partner who will provide constructive feedback. It is important to remember that levels of sensitivity differ between individuals. Learn from your partner's feedback and adjust your techniques appropriately.

Chapter Six will explain the basic hand application techniques that are used in Japanese foot massage. It is best to have a clear understanding of the differences in characteristics between each individual hand application technique before attempting to perform Japanese foot massage. Chapters Seven through Ten will introduce appropriate techniques for specific regions of the foot. These examples will help you to understand how to combine basic techniques in particular regions. For example, one technique may work well on the arch, but that same technique may not be appropriate on other parts of the foot. These differences must be mastered in order to determine which technique will be the most effective for a particular condition.

Understanding basic procedures and guidelines are the first steps in learning to perform Japanese foot massage. We will learn 60 different techniques, and you must practice each of them thoroughly before attempting a complete massage. A few general tips follow that will help you learn the application of a basic foot massage.

Tips for Getting Started

Japanese foot massage can be performed with a mat on the floor, in a reclining chair, or on a massage table. If using a massage table, you should adjust it properly (for guidelines see pp. 62 - 63). Additionally, the environment should be quiet, properly lit, and temperate. You can also add some relaxing music, if played softly.

Use your dominant hand when learning a new technique. If you are right-handed, practice the technique on the client's right foot. All of the examples in Chapters Seven through Ten are explained on the client's right foot. Once you become comfortable with the application of a technique using your dominant hand, reverse hand placements and practice on the other foot. Keep your shoulders down, elbows dropped, and wrists relaxed, except during a few pressure and vibration techniques which will require you to tense your muscles for a short period of time.

Performance Tips

Always start Japanese foot massage with warm up techniques. Warm up techniques should be applied lightly and smoothly. You can combine examples of the techniques in whatever order you wish. Whether you perform a stroking, kneading, or pressure technique, always begin by applying light force, gradually increasing it over the course of the massage .

A foot massage is always performed more quickly when using gentler force. As you apply more force, you must slow down your movements. At times, Japanese foot massage requires fast application to shake, relax, and loosen muscles. Sometimes fast stroking is used to make the movement feel continuous. All fast movements must be applied lightly and smoothly. Begin practicing slowly. Do not rush. If you rush, your client may have a difficult time relaxing. The speed of the technique will come naturally with practice and experience. Nver apply deep pressure with fast motion.

Special precautions must be taken when applying Japanese foot massage on infants, the elderly, or persons with injuries or illnesses. The amount of force must be eased and added very gradually. Perform massage more frequently, but for a shorter duration. For instance, substitute two sessions that are a ten minutes in length for a single session of twenty minutes. Some techniques may require modifications to fit the smaller feet of infants or children.

Japanese Foot Massage: Before and After

It is helpful to warm the foot with a moist heating pad or towel before and after the foot massage. The application of heat will increase circulation, rid the feet of toxins, and help your client relax. The temperature must be warm, and not too hot. Although it is preferable to use a heating device (such as a hydrocollator), heating up a wet towel in a crock pot may be substituted. Do not use an electric heating pad or blanket. Some clients have very thick, hard skin on the feet with hardly any sensitivity at all. Tough skin can be very difficult to work with. Soaking the client's feet in warm water for five to ten minutes will help loosen tougher skin.

Hydrocollators and related supplies are available.
See back of the book for details.

After the massage, wipe the feet with a dry towel, or steam the feet with a warm wet towel, and wipe them afterward. Warming the feet for two or three minutes is sufficient. Do not allow the towel to become chilled, as cold will decrease circulation in the feet and greatly reduce the benefits of a foot massage. You may advise the client to take a warm bath or sauna after the massage.

Drinking water after the treatment will help to eliminate toxins from the body. It is essential that your client drink about two cups of warm water. If your client has a heart, liver, or kidney disease, this amount should be reduced to about 3/4 of a cup of water. Tea, coffee, soda, or even juices are not suitable substitutes. Warm water is ideal, though water at room temperature is satisfactory. Cold water chills the internal organs and decreases circulation. If your client does not drink enough water, these toxins will stay in the bloodstream and the effects of the massage will be lessened.

Sometimes after a massage your client may feel some soreness for a day or two. Drinking plenty of water will reduce soreness, but a hot bath, whirlpool, or jacuzzi soon after the massage may also help.

Applications for those with Injuries or Surgery

If you have a client who has had recent surgery or has an injury, you may still be able to perform a massage. Apply the treatment cautiously without working directly on bruises, stitches, or broken skin.

Applications for those with Pain Throughout the Feet

Some feet are very sensitive to even a light amount of pressure. This does not necessarily mean that the entire body is in poor condition, or that the person is seriously ill. It it may mean only that the client has a low tolerance threshold for pain or pressure. In these situations, take extra time to warm the feet, then add gradual, gentle force. Generally, after several treatments, the tolerance threshold will be raised and you should be able to work normally.

Japanese Foot Massage and Lubrication

Most Japanese foot massage techniques that come from Zoku Shin Do require some form of lubrication. Oil, lotion, or a mixture of the two are most commonly used. If you are familiar with giving Swedish or other types of oil massage, these techniques should feel comfortable to you. If you are used to performing bodywork without oil, it will take some getting used to. I find that lotion is easier to handle, but try different combinations until you find what works best for you. Always ask your client first, before using fragrant oils or lotions, because some clients may have allergies or reactions to specific substances. Do not put the lubricant directly on the client, always warm the lubricant in your hands first.

> Various
> *Quality Foot Lubricants*
> are also available.
> *See back of the book*
> *for details.*

Duration and Frequency of Treatments

The duration of Japanese foot massage can be as short as two or three minutes, or as long as 20 minutes. It can be performed by itself, or as part of an entire body massage. The length of the massage will depend upon how much time is available, as well as the size, age, personal needs, and health conditions of your client.

The frequency of application is very important. The therapist must adjust the amount of massage application according to frequency. When determining the "dosage" of massage, consider the duration, as well as the correct pressure and location. Treatments should be performed consistently, both in terms of methods and frequency. Develop a regular schedule with your client, such as once or twice a week, or every ten days. It is much more effective to receive foot massage on a regular basis, rather than to receive several treatments within a short period of time and then goseveral months without treatment.

Generally, ten to twenty minutes is a comfortable amount of time for a Japanese foot massage. Massages of twenty minutes or more drain both the therapist and the client. If you are not able to complete a massage in one session, another visit should be arranged. While Japanese foot massage can be received daily, I do not recommend exceeding one session per day. Lifestyle changes or stress management may be suggested for a client who requires more than one session per day. One or two sessions per week is sufficient for most.

Combining Japanese Foot Massage with Other Massage

Japanese foot massage techniques can be easily incorporated into a full Anma, Shiatsu, or Western massage routine. You can also use these techniques as a warm up for either Western or Eastern reflexology, or to enhance a pedicure. When combining foot massage with other practices, a five to ten minute application is usually sufficient. Remember: always massage the feet **after** massaging the face.

Before Applying Japanese Foot Massage

I recommend following these simple guidelines before applying a massage:

1. To eliminate bacterial infections, keep your fingernails short.
2. Keep your hands clean. Wash them with anti-bacterial soap between each massage session.
3. Remove your watch and rings when applying a massage so that tendons in the wrist and fingers are not restricted.
4. Warm up, stretch, and massage your fingers, hands and arms.
5. Inquire if your client has had any injuries, surgery, and/or health problems.
6. Inquire if your client has any communicable diseases which you should be aware of, such as flu or tuberculosis.
7. Make sure to relax the client and yourself.
8. Make sure that your hands are warm for initial contact.

Your client should:

1. Clean the feet thoroughly before a massage.
2. Remove foot or ankle jewelry.
3. Wear comfortable clothes so that the feet are easily accessible.
4. Avoid being extremely hungry or extremely full during a treatment.
5. Drink water after the massage.
6. Rest and remain relaxed after a treatment.

Do not apply Japanese foot massage if the client suffers from:

1. A fever
2. A contagious illness
3. Having had recent surgery, especially on the feet
4. Skin infections

These are symptoms of contagious skin conditions or infections:

1. White patches on the bottoms of the feet, particularly if the feet are damp
2. Breakdown of the skin, including pitting on the surface
3. Raised bumps on the skin, sometimes looking similar to cauliflower
4. Peeling or cracked skin which may be red and inflamed
5. Any discoloration away from healthy and pink

Remember that you have the right to refuse any client a massage if you suspect a condition which could be contagious. Always wash with anti-bacterial soap before and immediately after treatment to reduce the risk of infections. Have your client consult a doctor if you or the client are in doubt about a medical condition.

Using and Developing the Thumb

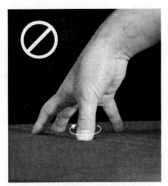

Rotating with the thumb joint

Japanese foot massage contains more finger manipulation than hand manipulation. This can exhaust the finger muscles or overwork the thumb. For the intensive techniques of Japanese foot massage, it is important to develop strength in your fingers, thumbs, and especially the muscles which support the thumbs. If you are not accustomed to using your thumb muscles, they will tire quickly and easily. To give the thumb recovery time during treatment, it helps to alternate techniques which use the thumb with applications that do not. Development of these muscles is one of the essential requirements for mastering Japanese foot massage. The best method for developing the thumb is to perform foot massage often.

Some Techniques to Avoid

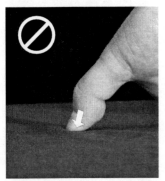

Pressure with a bent thumb

Many massage therapists complain of problems in the hands or fingers. One should always properly warm up the hands before working on a client. Stretch and massage your hands before and after applying Zoku Shin Do or Japanese foot massage, to keep them in the best possible working condition.

You should not have any stress, pain, or overstretched feelings in your hands, fingers, wrists, elbows, or shoulders while performing a massage. These sensations indicate incorrect application or positioning. You must check your hand application and readjust yourself to find the correct, comfortable position. Protecting yourself is the first priority. An injury built up over time can ruin a therapist's hands, and their practice as well. The following are some common mistakes made in applications and how to correct them.

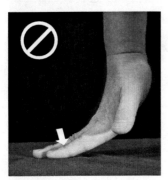

Hyperextending the fingers

1) Do not rotate with your thumb while applying heavy pressure (rotation from the metacarpals). This will cause significant wear on the thumb joints and cartilage. Instead, apply pressure with the thumb and use the rest of your hand to stabilize it. Rotate by using the whole hand from the shoulder, or from the elbow.

2) Do not apply pressure on the thumb when it is bent. Applying pressure when bending your thumb puts pressure on the joint instead of on the client. Keep the thumb straight and apply pressure perpendicularly to reduce stress, and to save premature wear on the joints.

3) Do not over bend the fingers backward to apply pressure. Instead, support the fingers by slightly rotating your wrist and placing adjacent fingers behind or alongside of each other.

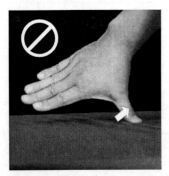

Hyperextending the thumb

4) Do not stroke or apply pressure with the side of the thumb, or allow it to hyperextend as you stroke, because it creates stress to the carpometacarpal and metacarpophalangeal joints. Change the angle of the thumb so that you push into the stroke with the hand.

Hand Maintenance Method:

As a massage therapist, especially at the professional level, it is very important that you properly maintain your hands. Many hand problems can be prevented, reduced, or eliminated by performing a daily maintenance massage on your own hands and forearms. When working for several hours at a time, it is essential that you massage and stretch your hands frequently. This is especially important when you feel tightness in your forearms and hands, a condition which often occurs the morning after a day of performing massage.

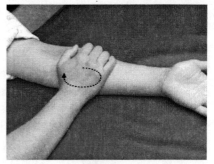
Palm rotation on the forearm

Make sure that you properly warm and loosen the muscles before performing a massage. Spend about five minutes stretching and massaging your fingers, hands, wrists, arms, and shoulders before and after each massage. I teach my students a routine of 25 techniques to maintain the hands. Here are four of the most important techniques.

1. Palm Rotation (Ju Netsu Ho) on the Forearm

Place your arm on the massage table with the palm up. Grasp the inner (medial) edge of the forearm with the palm of your other hand. Apply pressure into your forearm and rotate, using your entire shoulder and arm. Continue applying rotation to the entire forearm until it is warm.

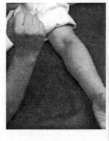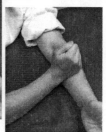
Percussion on the forearm

2. Percussion (Ko Da Ho) on the Forearm

Position your arm as you did in the previous technique. Make a loose fist with your other hand. Strike your forearm with the loose fist, keeping your wrist loose. You can strike with the front of your fist (as pictured), the side of your wrist, or the back of your hand. Again, cover your entire forearm.

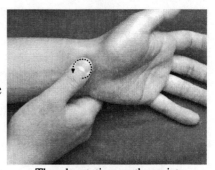
Thumb rotation on the wrist

3. Thumb Rotations (Ju Netsu Ho) on the Wrist

Place your thumb on the inner side of the wrist, just below the other thumb, and wrap the fingers around behind the wrist for support. Apply rotation by using your entire hand (not just the thumb). Move the thumb across the middle of the wrist, working your way to the inner side of the hand (hypothenar side) and repeat the rotation. Repeat the whole sequence on the other side of the wrist.

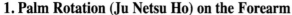
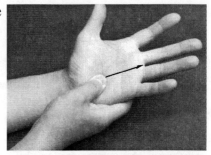
Stroking between the metacarpals

4. Stroking (Kei Satsu Ho) Between the Metacarpals

Place your thumb on the heel of your hand, wrapping the fingers behind the hand for support. Use the thumb to stroke slowly between the metacarpal bones. Begin just above the wrist, and end between the base of each finger. Work between all of the metacarpals (including between the thumb and index finger). Repeat stroking on the other side of the hand. Lubrication can be used if needed.

For further information:
*Hand Maintenance Guide
for Massage Therapists*
ISBN 1 - 57615 - 030 - 5
Kotobuki Publications
see back of this book for details.

Client Positioning for Japanese Foot Massage

Japanese foot massage can be applied in either the lay on the back (supine) position or the lay on the stomach (prone) position. It can be applied in other positions as well, such as on the side position, but these are rarely used. In Chapters Seven through Ten, 60 examples of techniques are demonstrated that show how to work in the lay on the back position. Chapter Eleven explains how to convert those techniques into the lay on the stomach position. Both have distinct characteristics and offer different advantages and disadvantages.

There are many ways to apply Japanese foot massage. A massage or salon table is often used, but not everybody has a table, and some people may prefer to work on the floor. A reclining chair can be used with some support under the calf, or the client can lay across a sofa with the leg resting on the arm of the sofa. There are several options, but it is important that you position yourself comfortably in relation to the foot, so that it is easier to apply Japanese foot massage and to minimize the stress to your body. Make sure that your client is positioned comfortably as well.

Japanese foot massage can be applied on a regular massage table, which should be sturdy and not squeak. It should be easy to adjust for different heights. Do not use extremely wide or narrow tables, because they make massage more difficult to apply (28 - 31 inches wide is ususally the best). The fabric should be water and oil resistant for easy cleaning and sanitizing between massages.

Regardless of whether you are working on a massage table or on the floor, there should be a sheet or cover between the client and the table (or floor). Using a twin size sheet under the client will work well for most tables. If you are working on a sofa or reclining chair, you should place a large towel under the foot to protect the fabric from lubricant. Make sure that the rest of the body is covered to warm the client. Sheets and towels must be changed between each massage.

The client's legs should be raised between six and twelve inches from the floor, with large cushions or pillows to bring them up to a comfortable working level (see p 96). A small pillow can be placed under the client's head for comfort, but do not raise the head too far. Do not raise the upper torso, because it will tilt the pelvis and lock the legs, making it difficult to apply some of the foot massage techniques.

A peaceful and quiet environment can enhance the massage as well. It is best to apply the massage in a warm and quiet room. Interruptions and noises, such as phone calls, should be reduced to a minimum. Soft, soothing music can also be added for relaxation.

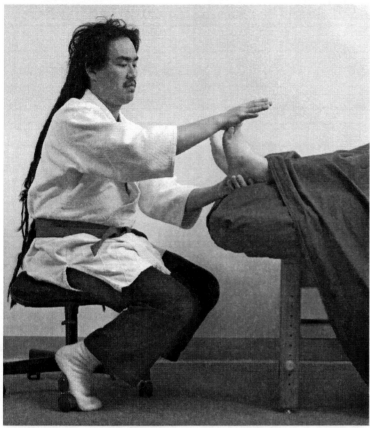

Japanese foot massage is most often applied on either a massage table or the floor. Chapter Eleven explains both settings for the lay on the stomach positions.

Massage Table Settings for Japanese Foot Massage

The Japanese foot massage techniques are designed, and have been modified, to be performed on a massage table set at a regular height. If you are using a salon style table, make sure that the client's entire lower legs and feet are raised so that they are level with the table from the knees to the feet. A massage table should not be set too high or too low. Sit on a chair at the end of the table and adjust the height so that the foot is level with your chest.

Applying Japanese Foot Massage on the Floor

Since Japanese foot massage is traditionally performed on the floor, the techniques work well without the use of a massage table. If you are combining Japanese foot massage with Anma, Shiatsu, or other bodywork, you will find that they will compliment each other.

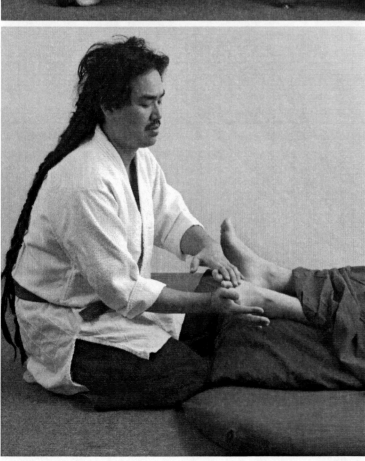

You can have your client lay on a thin futon, pad, or carpeted floor for comfort. Many westerners are not accustomed to kneeling for long periods of time. You can sit on a pillow or cushion for comfort. When working on the floor, it helps to raise the foot with a pillow or some other kind of support.

Chapter Six

THE BASIC TECHNIQUES OF JAPANESE FOOT MASSAGE

In this chapter, I introduce the hand manipulation techniques of Japanese foot massage. The majority of Japanese foot massage techniques came from Anma, and have been modified over a period of time to work specifically on the feet.

The many techniques of Japanese foot massage are divided into categories. Each category has its own unique character and purpose that will be explained in this chapter. It is important to have a clear understanding of the differences between the characteristics of each category of techniques. Memorizing these categories will make it much easier for you to differentiate between the dozens of techniques as you learn them.

Chapters Seven through Eleven provide examples of Japanese foot massage techniques to show how each is performed. To effectively learn Japanese foot massage, you must first learn each example of the technique individually. Initially, this may seem very fragmented, but it is very important to understand the qualities and purpose of each technique before stringing them together. Later in your training you will learn to combine them fluently to develop a smooth, coordinated massage.

For those of you familiar with Anma, I have included Japanese terminology for easy reference. It is not necessary to memorize these words in order to practice Japanese foot massage, nor is an understanding of Japanese language or culture needed to understand the techniques.

Japanese Foot Massage Application Techniques

Japanese foot massage application techniques are mainly derived from Anma. Anma is constructed of seven foundational categories of techniques:

1. Kei Satsu Ho   Light Stroking Techniques
2. Ju Netsu Ho   Kneading Techniques
3. Shin Sen Ho   Vibrating Techniques
4. Ap Paku Ho   Pressure Techniques
5. Ko Da Ho   Percussion Techniques
6. Kyoku Te Ho   Special Percussion Techniques
7. Un Do Ho   Movement, Stretching, and Exercise Techniques

The kneading technique, Ju Netsu Ho, is the primary technique used in Anma. In Japanese foot massage, the stroking technique, (Kei Satsu Ho), is the foundational technique. The kneading technique, (Ju Netsu Ho), the vibration technique (Shin Sen Ho), the pressure technique, (Ap Paku Ho), and the stretching technique, (Un Do Ho) are used together to enhance the effects of the massage.

Anma also has supplemental techniques which are used less often:

8. Kyo Satsu Ho   Stroking / Rotating Techniques with Heavy Pressure
9. Ha Aku Ho   Gripping and Squeezing Techniques
10. Ken Biki Ho   Pulling and Traction Techniques
11. Shin Kin Ho   Stretching the Muscles, Tendons, or Fascia

I will also briefly introduce five Shiatsu techniques in this chapter, although they are used infrequently. Because Shiatsu grew out of Anma, the nature of the techniques are very similar and overlap each other. Understanding Anma techniques is sufficient enough to be able to give Japanese foot massage.

Each individual technique is unique in character and offers different effects from all of the others. Combining different techniques will offer better and faster results than simply performing one technique repeatedly. As you progress in your practice of massage, you will develop a sense of how to efficiently combine techniques so as to offer the correct technique in the appropriate situation. As you begin combining techniques, select a few and try to smoothly alternate between them. You will eventually learn to make only marginal changes in the amount of force and speed used in each technique.

For further information about the application of Japanese Massage techniques, refer to the book:

ANMA: The Art of Japanese Massage

See back of this book for details.

Another reason for combining techniques is that different techniques require the use of different muscles in your hand. By frequently alternating between techniques, you can avoid over-exerting one particular part of the hand. Also, the muscles that are used for movement during application are less likely to tire.

How to Understand the Japanese Characters of Techniques

Throughout this book I have included the Japanese names of the hand manipulation techniques for each example. Although it is not necessary to memorize all of these names, you should memorize at least the names of the basic techniques and pressure points if you are serious about your Japanese foot massage practice. To advance in the study of any traditional Japanese medicine, it is important for Westerners to understand the rudiments of the native language. It has been my experience that most of my students enjoy learning and understanding the names and technical language of Japanese foot massage, Anma, and Shiatsu.

Below is an example which shows how common Japanese foot massage and Anma techniques are named in Japanese.

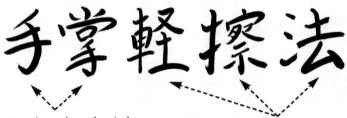

The first two (sometimes three) characters show which part of the hand the massage is applied with. In this case, Sho Ko indicates the entire palm.

The next three characters explain which technique is being applied. The last character is always "Ho" which means "technique". This example shows Kei Satsu Ho, a light stroking technique.

The entire set of characters means— "a light stroking technique applied with the entire palm". Below are some examples of the first two or three characters that indicate which part of the hand is used to apply the appropriate technique.

 Sho Ko

Sho Ko means "entire palm of the hand". Generally, it includes the insides of the fingers and the sides of the thumbs.

 Bo Shi

Bo means "mother" and Shi means "finger". Together, they have come to mean thumb. Bo Shi usually refers to the inside of the thumb.

 Bo Shi To

Bo Shi means "thumb" and To means the "tip" or "head", so Bo Shi To is the tip of thumb.

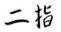 **Ni Shi**

Ni Shi means "the flat parts of two fingers". Normally, Ni Shi will refer to the index and middle fingers, but it can also refer to other combinations of two fingers

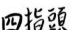 **Shi Shi To**

Shi Shi means "four fingers" and To means "tip" or "head", so Shi Shi To means "the tips of the four fingers".

 Shu Ken

Shu Ken means "hand-staff", and includes the top of the middle phalanges, the distal phalanges, or the top of the metacarpophalangeal and the interphalangeal joints.

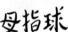 **Bo Shi Kyu**

Bo Shi means "thumb" and Kyu means "ball" so this is the thenar (radial carpal ball) region of the inner hand.

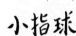 **Ko Shi Kyu**

Ko Shi means "pinky" and Kyu means "ball" so this is the hypothenar region of the outer hand (ulnar carpal ball).

 Shu Kon

Shu Kon refers to the region directly over the carpal bones which form the heel of the hand.

1. Light Stroking Technique - Kei Satsu Ho

軽擦法

Kei Satsu Ho

按撫法

also known as An Bu Ho

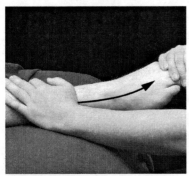

Shu Ko Kei Satsu Ho

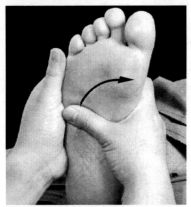

Bo Shi Kei Satsu Ho

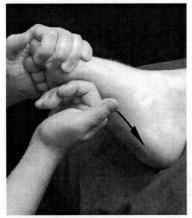

Shi Ka Kei Satsu Ho

Light stroking technique, or in Japanese, Kei Satsu Ho, is performed by sliding over the surface with either up-and-down or circular motions. This is one of the most common techniques of Anma and one of the primary techniques used in Japanese foot massage, especially when using lubrication. The light stroking is used to gently bring up heat to the surface of the area, relax muscles, and improve circulation.

In Anma, Kei Satsu Ho is most often performed without lubrication, but in Japanese foot massage it is often applied with lubrication. Regardless, it is very important to bring the heat to the surface and maintain the heat during the movement, especially when the application moves from one area to another.

Light stroking technique can be applied with various parts of the hand that are usually chosen for the best fit to both the parts of the body and purpose of technique. I will list most of the major ones that are commonly used for stroking the feet. The techniques most often used in Japanese foot massage are:

1) Stroking with the entire hand
   (Shu Ko Kei Satsu Ho)
2) Stroking with the flat part of the thumb
   (Bo Shi Kei Satsu Ho)
3) Stroking with the tip of the thumb
   (Bo Shi To Kei Satsu Ho)
4) Stroking with the base of the thumb - thenar
   (Bo Shi Kyu Kei Satsu Ho)
5) Stroking with the side of the hand - hypothenar
   (Ko Shi Kyu Kei Satsu Ho)
6) Stroking with the flat parts of four fingers
   (Shi Shi Kei Satsu Ho)
7) Stroking with the back of the fingers
   (Shi Ka Kei Satsu Ho)
8) Stroking with the top of the fist or knuckle
   (Shu Ken Kei Satsu Ho)

Here are some important tips and precautionary notes that you should know. Your wrists, elbows, and shoulders must be relaxed and loose enough to easily adjust to the contours of the feet and legs. Tense shoulders and elbows make for a jerky and uncomfortable application. You can increase the pressure of the stroking after the tissue is properly warmed, but do not use extreme pressure with this technique. Stroking must be applied smoothly and rhythmically. Your fingers must be kept together to ensure that the heat is kept on the surface of the skin.

2. Kneading Technique - Ju Netsu Ho

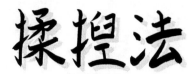

Ju Netsu Ho

also known as Ju Nen Ho

Kneading technique, or in Japanese, Ju Netsu Ho, is the primary technique used in Anma, but it is less often used in Japanese foot massage. This is because the application of Ju Netsu Ho is limited when you are unable to grasp the surface, and when lubricant is used it becomes even more difficult to apply. If you are accustomed to applying the kneading techniques of Swedish massage, these techniques might seem similar, but they are actually very different.

The main purpose of Ju Netsu Ho is to reduce the tension of the muscles and tendons. The two primary application types of Ju Netsu Ho are kneading and rotating. Kneading is usually applied through the continuous motion of squeezing and releasing the muscle between your fingers and the thumb or palm, similar to kneading bread dough. Rotation is applied by hooking a portion of the hand to the surface and applying circular motions without sliding over the skin. When you are kneading or rotating, it is very important that you pay close attention to the condition of the muscles to detect any kind of irregular tightness.

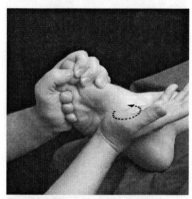

Bo Shi Kyu Ju Netsu Ho

There are many different ways to apply Ju Netsu Ho, including techniques which do not contain kneading or rotating movements. For example, you can knead by pushing the muscle between two alternating thumbs, or using very small, alternating strokes with the edges of the thumbs, both of which are demonstrated in this book.

The following are the Ju Netsu Ho applications most often used in Japanese foot massage:

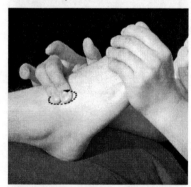

Ni Shi To Ju Netsu Ho

1) Kneading with the base of the thumb - thenar
   (Bo Shi Kyu Ju Netsu Ho)
2) Kneading with the side of the hand - hypothenar
   (Ko Shi Kyu Ju Netsu Ho)
3) Kneading with the flat part of the thumb
   (Bo Shi Ju Netsu Ho)
4) Kneading with the tip of the thumb
   (Bo Shi To Ju Netsu Ho)
5) Kneading with the tips of two fingers
   (Ni Shi To Ju Netsu Ho)

Ju Netsu Ho is not usually applied during warm up because it stimulates the muscles too deeply. It is less often used in techniques applied with lubricant (Chapters Seven and Eight), but it becomes a primary technique when working without lubricant (Chapter Nine).

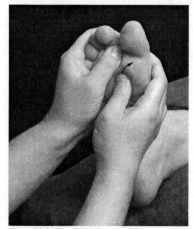

Bo Shi To Ju Netsu Ho

3. Vibration Technique - Shin Sen Ho

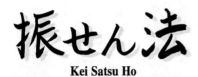

Kei Satsu Ho

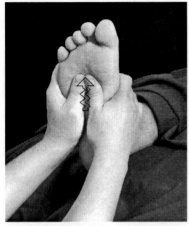

Bo Shi Shin Sen Ho

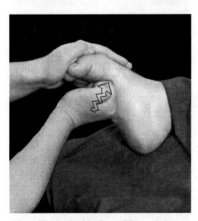

Shu Ken Shin Sen Ho

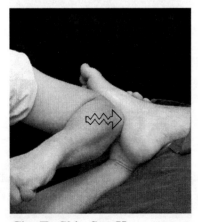

Chu To Shin Sen Ho

Vibration technique, or in Japanese, Shin Sen Ho, may sound simple, but developing fine control in your palms and fingers takes time and practice. This can be the most difficult technique to master. Proficiency can take years of practice, but your ability will improve as your hand skills develop.

Unlike stroking or kneading techniques that work on the surface, vibration aims to work deeper into the muscle. Practitioners often alternate between vibration and kneading. The combination has two benefits: they will loosen muscles more effectively, and the hands will not tire as quickly. Shin Sen Ho is also often combined with Ap Paku Ho (pressure technique, see next page). If a client finds that Ap Paku Ho is a little painful, vibration can be used to disperse the painful pressure over a larger area of muscle.

There are two different ways to apply vibration: inner and outer. The distinction between them lies not in the position of the hand, but in the type of movement you use to vibrate. The two techniques have different purposes, and it is important that you develop control of the depth, length, and speed of the vibrations. As with Ju Netsu Ho, some practice is required to master this technique.

I. Inner vibration 内振

With inner vibration, the point is to send fine, concentrated vibrational force into the inner layers of the muscle. Inner vibration is usually applied by tensing the entire upper body and sending the vibration from deep within your body. There should be little vibrational movement at the point of contact.

II. Outer vibration 外振

Outer vibration is used to loosen muscles on the surface of an area. While applying outer vibration, your upper body should remain loose and relaxed. Outer vibration is usually applied by using vigorous vibrations at the place of contact, and does not require the same level of concentration or vibrational force as inner vibration does.

Due to the shape of the feet, only a few vibrations work well.

1) Vibration with the thumb   (Bo Shi Shi Sen Ho)
2) Vibration with the fist   (Shu Ken Shin Sen Ho)
3) Vibration with the forearm (Zen Wan Sen Ho)

4. Pressure Technique - Ap Paku Ho

Pressure technique, or in Japanese, Ap Paku Ho, can be of any weight or duration, and can be applied in many different ways. Ap Paku Ho is very similar to O Atsu Ho — the primary pressure technique in Shiatsu. Anma practitioners who specialized in this technique early in the century began calling themselves Shiatsu therapists.

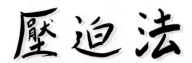

Strength of Pressure (Meli and Kali)

The amount of force you apply requires you to change the angle of your thumb in relation to the surface of the body. With heavy pressure, you must be closer to the fingertip in order to support a much more defined pressure, while a flat thumb is softer and does not require this support. Meli and Kali are the Japanese terms used to describe the different types of pressure used in Japanese foot massage.

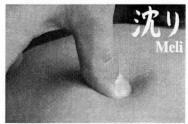

Meli literally means "sink" in Japanese. It uses the tip of the thumb (or fingers) to deeply sink into the skin. Meli is usually deep, heavy pressure for shorter durations, used in conjunction with breathing, and is often used for sedation (Sha in Japanese, see p. 27) with fewer deep, long applications.

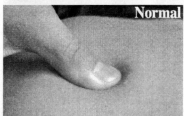

Kali literally means "floating" in Japanese. It uses light pressure with a flat finger or fingers held parallel to the skin surface. Kali is usually of longer duration with more frequent applications. The breathing cycle is not as important. It is often used for tonification (Ho in Japanese, see p. 27).

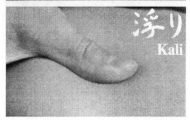

Open

Applying Pressure to the Acupoints (Tsubo)

This method is only used to stimulate the acupoints on the meridians (Kei Ketsu in Japanese, see p 32), in order to tonify or sedate the meridians. You must pay attention to the client's breathing cycle when applying pressure to the Kei Ketsu. As you press a tsubo, imagine three steps. First, imagine *opening* the tsubo with light pressure to make the body aware that you are going to stimulate it. Then, imagine entering *into* that tsubo as you press. This step requires strong pressure over a longer duration of time to stimulate the tsubo. Finally, imagine *closing* the tsubo using slightly lighter pressure for the same duration as the previous step. Closing is very important because it ensures that the tsubo is not left exposed.

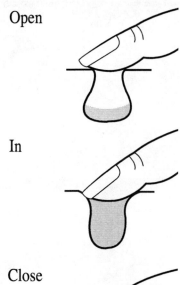

In

Close

5. Percussion Technique - Ko Da Ho

叩打法

Ko Da Ho

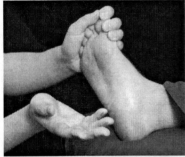

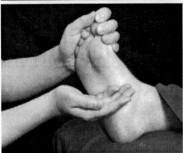

Setsu Da Ho

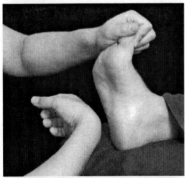

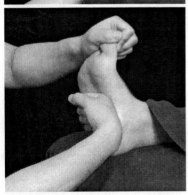

Shu Hai Ko Da Ho

Percussion or tapping techniques, in Japanese, Ko Da Ho, are not hitting techniques. It is usally applied with a loose wrist so that it does not feel like hitting. Anma has two percussion techniques: standard (Ko Da Ho) and special (Kyoku Te Ho). In Japan, Ko Da Ho are the best known techniques among laypersons and families, because percussion techniques are among the most fundamental and easiest to learn.

Ko Da Ho is applied rapidly and lightly by tapping the feet with different parts of your hand. The hand retains the same shape during the percussion, but your shoulder and elbow must be fairly loose and flexible. Percussion is usually applied by alternating both hands, but it can be applied with just one hand for application on the foot.

Ko Da Ho stimulates the feet deeper than other Japanese foot massage techniques. Other techniques such as kneading or stroking tend to affect only the surface of the foot, but percussion can stimulate the deepest layers of the tissue.

Because of the size and shape of the feet, only a few types of percussion are effective. Ko Da Ho works well for the bottom (plantar) of the foot, but it does not work well for the top (dorsal) of the foot, since the skin and bones are so close together. These are the techniques that will work well on the bottom of the foot:

1) Sides of closed hands   (Shu Ken Ko Da Ho)
2) Sides of open hands   (Setsu Da Ho)
3) Flat parts of the fingers (Shi Shi Ko Da Ho)
4) Tips of the fingers   (Shi To Ko Da Ho)
5) Bent hand   (Shu Ko Ko Da Ho)
6) Back of the hand   (Shu Hai Ko Da Ho)

Begin by practicing these techniques slowly until they are smooth and rhythmic. Try to get into a triplet rhythm, where you are skipping the second beat. The key is to be able to control your hands whether you are using hard or soft bounces. It is important to develop senses that will allow you to adjust to your clients' requirements. This should not be applied too forcefully, but just enough to be effective. You should eventually develop a sense of how much force to apply.

6. Special Percussion Technique - Kyoku Te Ho

Special percussion technique, or in Japanese, Kyoku Te Ho, is similar to Ko Da Ho, but is a unique way to perform percussion that is found only in Anma. The difference between the two is that Ko Da Ho is simple percussion, where the hand does not change shape during the application. Kyoku Te Ho is a series of specially modified percussion techniques where the hand changes shape during each percussive movement. Also, Kyoku Te Ho is typically a more gentle technique than Ko Da Ho. Kyoku Te Ho requires a fair amount of practice for smooth integration into the other techniques.

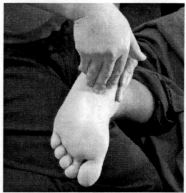

Unlike most other Japanese foot massage techniques, many Kyoku Te Ho techniques are only designed to work in specific regions of the body. While there are many variations of Kyoku Te Ho, only a few of these can be applied specifically on the feet.

Most often, Kyoku Te Ho is performed on the feet with the client in the prone position. Improper application of Kyoku Te Ho can create severe stress to the joints on your fingers or wrists. Proper training is highly recommended for a better understanding of Kyoku Te Ho. Due these circumstances, this edition of the book does not introduce any of Kyoku Te Ho. For students who have trained in Anma, I have listed below six of the most common and easiest variations that can be applied to the foot.

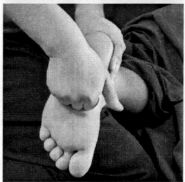

Kuruma Te

1) Fingertip striking then collapsing   (Tsuki Te)
2) Rolling knuckles   (Kuruma Te)
3) Collapsing the thumb   (Kujiki Te)
4) Quick pulling   (Yobi Te)
5) Sweeping   (Hajiki Te)
6) Two-handed paddle wheel inward   (Sukui Te)
7) Thumb and finger flipping   (Mawashi Te)

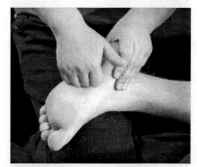

Kyoku Te Ho can add a special flavor to a masaage, but it is not a primary technique, and Japanese foot massage can be performed without it. It is usually only applied for specific conditions.

For more information about the application of Kyoku Te Ho techniques, please refer to Chapter 4 of *Anma: The Art of Japanese Massage*.

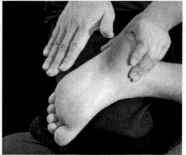

Hajiki Te

7. Stretch and Movement Technique - Un Do Ho

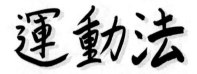

Stretch and movement techniques, or in Japanese, Un Do Ho, are a series of techniques which involve movement, stretching, and exercise. These are considered slightly advanced techniques, and while none of Un Do Ho techniques are immediately recognized as massage-like, they are still categorized as a part of massage techniques. Un Do Ho is an important part of Anma and Japanese foot massage because, when used in combination with the other techniques, it greatly enhances the therapeutic value of the treatment.

These techniques are commonly used in Japan for rehabilitation of injuries, and Un Do Ho is one of the oldest known techniques for rehabilitation. Modern Japanese rehabilitation techniques grew out of this tradition.

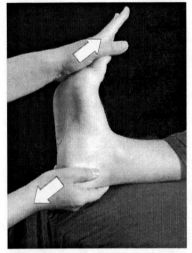

Shin Cho Un Do Ho

The purpose of movement and stretching is slightly different than the goals of other foot massage techniques. Each individual technique in Un Do Ho has a different purpose from the others. Stretching the muscles, aligning the structure, and regaining or maintaining the range of motion of the joint are the usual goals.

The majority of Un Do Ho techniques can generally be categorized into five different groups of techniques. These are:

1) movement by the client alone
   (Ji Do Un Do Ho)
2) adjustment techniques
   (Kyo Sei Ho)
3) movement by the therapist
   (Ta Do Un Do Ho)
4) stretching techniques
   (Shin Cho Un Do Ho)
5) exercising movement through resistance
   (Tei Ko Un Do Ho)

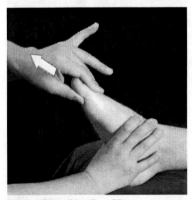

Shin Cho Un Do Ho

Un Do Ho must be applied very carefully and gently. Most of the techniques require you to work slowly as well. It is also very important to incorporate your client's breathing cycle into the application. Some techniques are advanced, and require classroom instruction and a solid understanding of anatomy and physiology. Because of this, only the Shin Cho Un Do Ho and Ta Da Un Do Ho are introduced in Chapter 10 of this book.

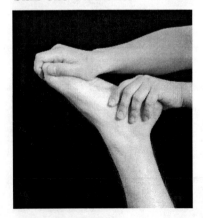

Ta Do Un Do Ho

The previous seven techniques are the traditional Anma techniques. Traditionally, Anma is known as containing seven application techniques, but in reality, there are many techniques in Anma that do not belong to this category. A few of these I have listed below as supplemental techniques.

8. Kyo Satsu Ho

Stroking/rotating technique with heavy pressure, or in Japanese, Kyo Satsu Ho, is like Kei Satsu Ho with heavy pressure. It is also called An Netsu Ho. Kyo Satsu Ho has two ways that it can be applied. Small rotations can be applied to the joint with heavy pressure, or you can stroke with heavy pressure using the thumb. Kyo Satsu Ho is not a commonly used technique, but it is usually applied to reduce pain and stiffness, as well as improve mobility of the joints.

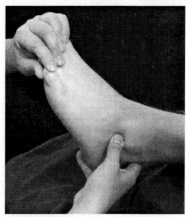

Bo Shi To Kyo Satsu Ho

9. Ha Aku Ho

Squeezing or grabbing technique, or in Japanese, Ha Aku Ho, is generally combined with other techniques such as stroking, vibration, or rotating to aid in the application. For example, Ha Aku Ho and Kei Satsu Ho can be combined to become Ha Aku Kei Satsu Ho (stroking while squeezing). Ha Aku Ho is not often used alone to work on the feet. The difference between Ha Aku Ho and Ap Paku Ho is that Ha Aku Ho squeezes from two directions simultaneously and Ap Paku Ho applies pressure from only one direction.

10. Ken Biki Ho

Pulling and applying tension technique, or in Japanese, Ken Biki Ho, is rarely used by itself on the feet. It is generally used to lightly stretch by pulling or to apply tension to the muscle in combination with another technique for enhanced effects.

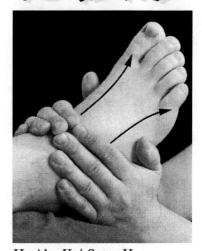

Ha Aku Kei Satsu Ho

11. Shin Kin Ho

Special stretching technique, or in Japanese, Shin Kin Ho, is particularly useful for application on smaller regions where you must manually force the muscles, tendons, or fascia to stretch or break adhesions in the tissues. It is usually applied to regions with limited mobility that are difficult to stretch.

12. Shiatsu Techniques

Most of the techniques used in Japanese Foot Massage are from Anma, but a few of them are derived from Shiatsu. Shiatsu was developed in the early 1900's and was categorized as a method of Anma until 1964, when Shiatsu became independent of Anma. Since Shiatsu developed from Anma, most Shiatsu techniques are very similar to Anma, and large portions of the applications overlap each other.

The techniques themselves may have similarities between them, yet the method of application is quite different. The primary difference between Anma and Shiatsu is that Anma is a kneading-based therapy, and Shiatsu is a pressure-based therapy. While Anma combines a diverse range of techniques, Shiatsu primarily uses pressure applications and seldom uses other techniques.

The following five techniques are used in modern Shiatsu practice.

1) O Atsu Ho
Push and pressure technique, or in Japanese, O Atsu Ho, is the pressure technique of Shiatsu. It is the same technique as Ap Paku Ho of Anma, but tends to rely more on the thumb.

2) An Netsu Ho
This technique is identical to Kyo Satsu Ho of Anma, but Shiatsu practitioners call it An Netsu Ho.

3) Shin Do Ho
This is a vibration technique used in Shiatsu. In Anma, it is called Shin Sen Ho. They are the same technique, although more pressure is usually applied with Shin Do Ho.

4) Bu Satsu Ho
This is technically the same as Kei Satsu Ho from Anma although it is usually applied with slightly more pressure. It is commonly used in the abdomen.

5) Shin Ten Ho
This is a stretching technique used in Shiatsu. It is identical to Ta Do Un Do Ho and Shin Cho Un Do Ho of the Un Do Ho techniques in Anma.

Meanings of the symbols used in this book

To accompany the written explanation, I have placed several types of arrows over the pictures to help visually explain different types of movement. The different types of arrows show different types of movement or pressure made while applying Japanese foot massage. Being familiar with the signs listed below will aid you in understanding this book.

Bold straight arrows

These arrows show the direction of stroking that slides over the surface of the skin. This arrow mainly indicates Kei Satsu Ho or Kyo Satsu Ho.

Dotted straight arrows

These arrows show the direction of pressure or movement that grips skin and muscle, which way to pull or push, or just the direction of applied pressure for techniques such as Ju Netsu Ho, Ap Paku Ho, and Ha Aku Ho. The dotted arrow means that your hands should remain in the same position relative to the skin, and not move over the skin.

Bold circular arrows

These show the direction of circular stroking, mainly in the case of Kei Satsu Ho. This movement slides over the skin or the clothes.

Dotted circular arrows

These arrows show the direction of rotation or circular movement that grips the muscle or skin, without moving over the skin. Your hand moves just slightly in the direction of the applied pressure such as with Ju Netsu Ho and Kyo Satsu Ho. The three-quarter and some of the half circles show continuing rotation. The one-quarter and the rest of the half circular arrows show movement. Refer to the instructions in the text for each case.

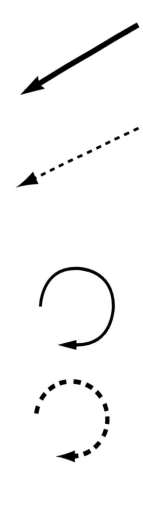

Zig zag arrows

These arrows show vibration. The direction of the arrow shows the direction of the pressure you should apply with the vibration.

Three dimensional arrows

These show movement of the body. This arrow is also used to indicate a direction of pressure that could be difficult to demonstrate with a two-dimensional arrow.

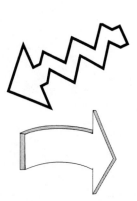

Chapter Seven

JAPANESE FOOT MASSAGE
WARM UP TECHNIQUES

In this chapter, I will introduce fifteen examples of Japanese foot massage warm up techniques. Warm up techniques are light, smooth movements to improve circulation, relax the muscles of the feet, as well as relax the client. They also prepare the feet for the deeper, more stimulating work that I will discuss in the next few chapters. Warm up techniques are usually used to begin a treatment, but they are also often used as a break between techniques, or to finish the massage with a smooth, light touch.

I will demonstrate these techniques on the right foot because many people are right-handed and find it easier to learn applications on the client's right foot. Apply the warm up techniques to the right foot and then repeat them on the left, or apply the techniques of all four chapters to the right and then to the left. All of the techniques in this and the following chapter are demonstrated with lubricants. Lotion, oil, or a combination of the two work well.

After learning all fifteen techniques, connect them in a sequence to compose a full warm up massage. These fifteen techniques can be performed in any order and repeated as often as you desire. Try not to break contact while thinking about which technique to do next in the sequence. Continue performing a given technique until you remember which one comes next. It is important to practice smooth transitions between techniques.

If your time is limited, you can combine the warm up techniques with a few selected examples from other chapters to address the client's needs. This brief massage should be sufficient for most clients if you are unable to do a more complete treatment.

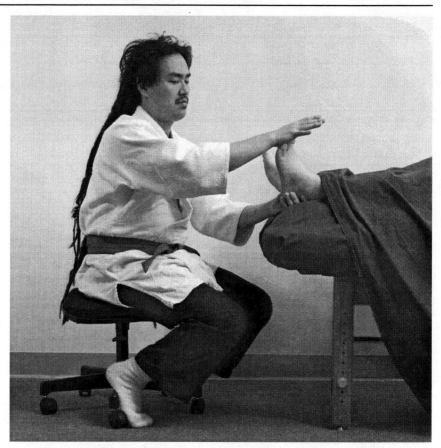

Apply on the table - Lay on the back (supine) position :

People who practice massage often use massage tables. If your client is lying on a massage table, you can sit (or kneel) at the end of the table as shown in the picture above. The client's feet should be placed roughly 2 to 6 inches from the end of the table.

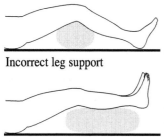

Incorrect leg support

Correct leg support

Japanese foot massage leg support cushions, massage tables, special foot lubrication, and a complete line of massage supplies are available. See back of this book for details or call 1-800-651-2662.

It is very important that the angle of the foot be as upright as possible to minimize stress to your wrists and shoulders. It is best to find a large cushion to raise the entire lower half of the legs so that the feet are level with the top of the chest. Completely raising the lower legs will also help reduce stress to the client's lower back. For this sort of massage it is not good to support the underside of the knees with a conventional bolster. This tilts the feet downward, making it difficult to work.

If you do not have large cushions to support the entire lower leg, it is better not to use any support at all. Instead, lower your chair to adjust yourself properly. If you feel any stress in your thumbs or wrists, adjust the positioning of the client's feet. It is better not to give the massage if the angle of the feet is stressful to your wrists because it can lead to pain and wrist problems. Of course, your arms and shoulders should remain relaxed as well.

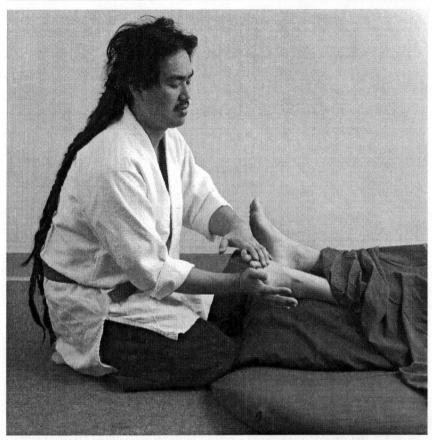

Apply on the floor - Lay on the back (supine) position :

Most people do not own a massage table. If you do not, don't worry-
-Japanese foot massage can be easily performed on the floor, on a
mat, or on a futon. Working on the floor is the way that massage has
been given in Japan for centuries. Many professional therapists who
practice an East Asian based massage such as Anma, Shiatsu, or Tui-
na, still prefer to work on the floor. Sit on your knees (seiza position) at the end of the mat, as shown in the picture above. If you
experience discomfort in this position you can sit on a small pillow.
I recommend that you avoid sitting cross-legged because it is more
difficult to use heavier pressure. If you do not have a mat or a massage table, or are uncomfortable on the floor, you can have the client
sit on a fully reclined chair (with foot support) or on a couch with
their legs supported by one of the arms.

Again, make sure to raise and support the client's lower legs so that
their toes are pointed straight up in the air. It is even more critical to
have the client's feet in the air when you work on the floor because it
is not possible to lower your body position in a chair or by crouch-
ing. Add extra pillows if needed, to raise yourself or to be more
comfortable. You may also place another pillow behind the client's
shoulders and head for their comfort.

Japanese Foot Massage Techniques - Example #1

Light Stroking on the Feet and Legs

Japanese name of this technique

手掌軽擦法

Shu Ko Kei Satsu Ho

The purpose of this technique

Increase circulation to the foot and relax the client

Where it is applied

Over the shin bones, ankles and feet

About this technique

Begin the Japanese foot massage with this long stroking technique. It will increase circulation to the entire foot and legs, and will also help to relax the client. Make sure that your strokes are very smooth, light, fairly quick, and maintain even pressure. Use one hand at a time.

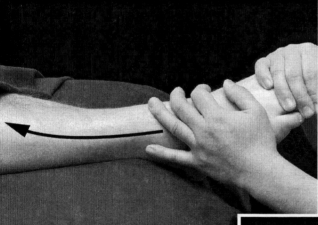

Stroking the outside of the shin:

1 Gently place your inner (right) hand (see p 20) on the toes to flatten and stabilize the foot. Keep your elbow relaxed and dropped so that your arm supplies the needed light pressure.

2 Place the palm of your outer (left) hand on the top (dorsal) of the foot with your fingers at a 45° angle to the shin bone.

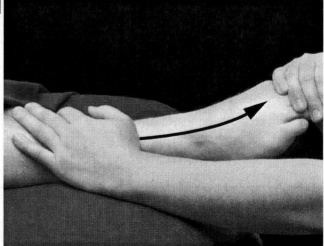

3 With plenty of lubrication (a hairy leg will require lots), stroke the foot and leg with the palm and the bottom half of your fingers of your outer hand. Stroke past the ankle and over the shin bone (fibula) to just below the knee and back down again to the toes. Keep your hand flat and at a 45° angle to the shin bone during the entire stroke. Repeat 10 - 15 times.

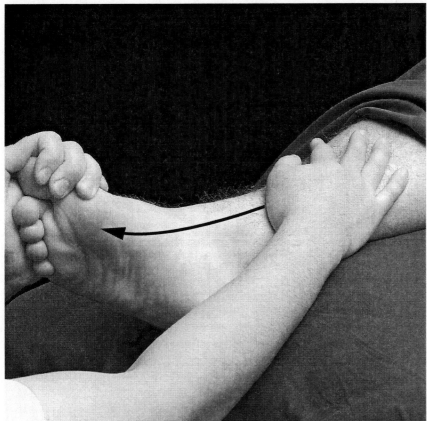

Stroking the inside of the foot:

4 Use your outer hand to grasp the foot around the big toe and slightly rotate the foot outward to have better access to the inside (medial side) of the leg.

5 Using your inner hand, stroke the area between the shin bone and the calf (gastrocnemus) muscle. Make sure that the fingers are pointed at a 45° angle to the bone and remain at that angle while stroking the entire leg and foot.

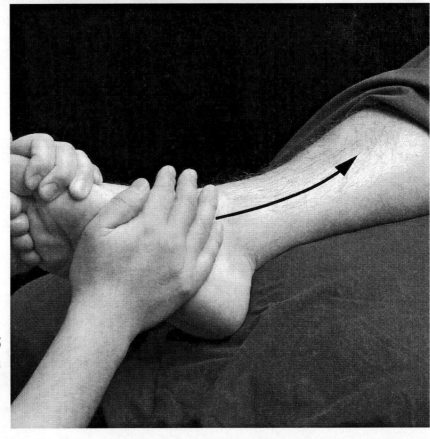

6 Stroke up and down from the sole of the foot to just below the knee 10 - 15 times. Beginning with step 1, repeat the entire sequence on the other foot.

Japanese Foot Massage Techniques - Example #2

Light Stroking on the Feet

Japanese name of this technique:

手掌軽擦法

Shu Ko Kei Satsu Ho

The purpose of this technique

Increase circulation of the foot

Where it is applied

On the top and bottom (dorsal and plantar) sides of the feet

About this technique

This is a fast-stroking technique which is used to warm and relax the feet. Applications should only last a short period of time or your hands will tire. You may find it easier to apply this technique if you move your body laterally to the corner of the table. This can help relieve potential stress to your wrists.

Stroking along the foot:

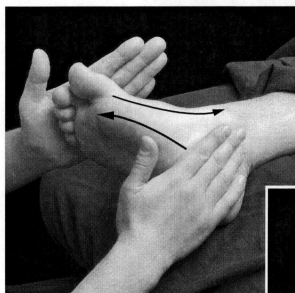

1 Place the foot between your hands and point the fingers toward the ceiling. Your outer (left) hand should be on top of the toes. The inner (right) hand should be over the heel. Make sure to have a sufficient amount of lubrication on your hands for smooth stroking.

2 Stroke rapidly back and forth along the arch and the top (dorsal) of the foot, alternating the direction of your hands to keep the strokes opposite from each other. Make sure that the foot is moving from the ankle with your hands to help smooth the movement. Cover the entire arch and top of the foot.

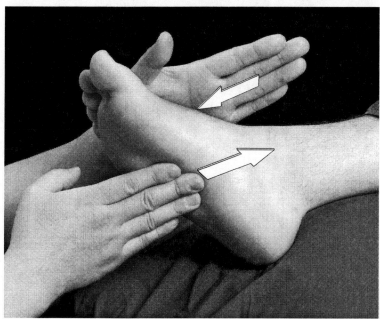

Stroking across the foot:

3 Place the foot between your hands with the fingers angled 45° inward. Your hands should be directly opposite each other (instead of on opposite ends of the foot as in the previous example). Alternate the direction of each stroke using the entire palm and fingers to move quickly, vigorously and smoothly back and forth across the foot. This should feel similar to lathering up a bar of soap.

4 Move up and down the foot from the edge of the heel pad to the base of the toes. Do not continue onto the toes because you may scratch yourself on the client's toenails. Again, make sure to use a sufficient amount of lubrication for smoother strokes. Continue for 30 - 45 seconds using both variations, then repeat on the other foot.

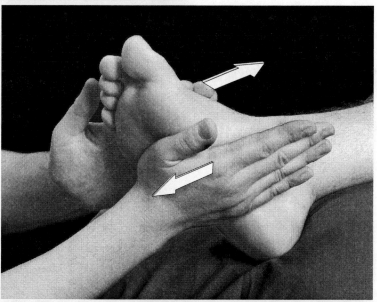

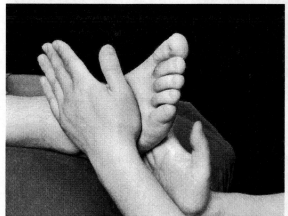

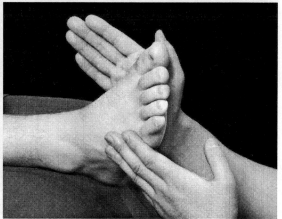

These are outer views of the foot for this technique.

Japanese Foot Massage Techniques - Example #3

Light Stroking Across the Feet

Japanese name of this technique:

手掌軽擦法

Shu Ko Kei Satsu Ho

The purpose of this technique

Increase the circulation and relax the foot

Where it is applied

Top and bottom (dorsal and plantar) sides of the feet

About this technique

This is another technique for warming the feet. Use rapid, back and forth strokes with enough lubrication for smooth movements. When applying this technique, it is very important that your wrist and elbow are relaxed so that your stroking is smooth.

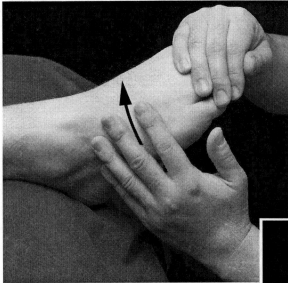

Straight stroking on the top (dorsal) of the foot:

1 Gently rest your inner (right) hand on the toes to flatten and stabilize the foot by letting your elbow relax and sink. Place the palm of your outer (left) hand on the top (dorsal) of the foot with the fingers pointed inward (medially). Start stroking with the fingers of your outer hand and then up over the top of the foot with the entire palm.

2 Stroke back to the outside (lateral) edge of the foot. Repeat the movement by stroking in both directions rapidly. Repeat 10 - 15 times, moving your hand between the toes and the ankle to cover the entire region on the top of the foot.

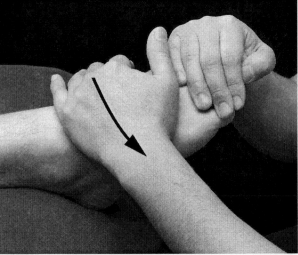

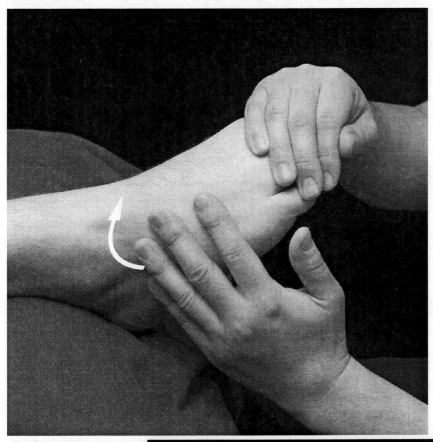

Circular stroking on the top (dorsal) of the foot:

3 Keep the same hand position for the inner hand as in step 1. Place the palm of your outer hand on the top of the foot with the fingers pointed inward and resting near the arch.

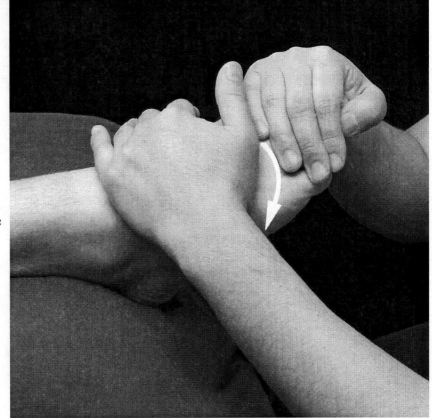

4 Stroke in a circular manner around the top of the foot with the palm of your hand. Use the fingertips as a pivot point as you stroke in a circle. Repeat 10 - 15 times. You can combine both straight and circular stroking techniques to smoothly cover the entire top of the foot.

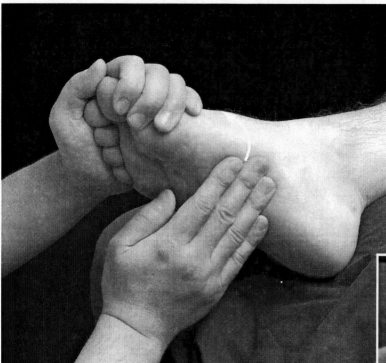

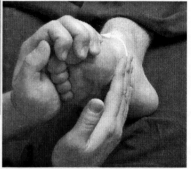

Straight stroking on the arch of the foot:

5 Use your outer hand to grasp around the big toe. Place the fingertips of the inner hand on the arch. Stroke by moving up the arch from your fingertips to your palm. Use plenty of lubrication so that the stroke remains smooth.

6 Bend your hand and fingers as you stroke. Do not stroke over to the top (dorsal) of the foot. Use the fingertips to stabilize as you stroke with your palm. Once the heel of the hand reaches the inner (medial) edge of the foot, reverse direction back to the starting position. Thoroughly work the arch by stroking back and forth 10 - 15 times.

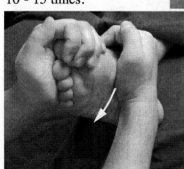

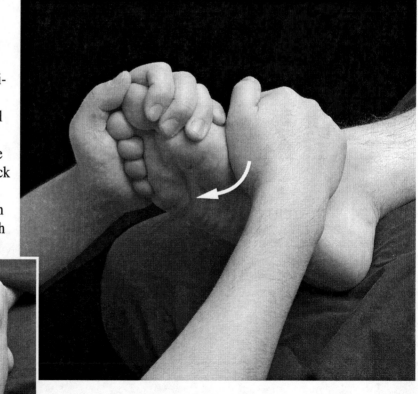

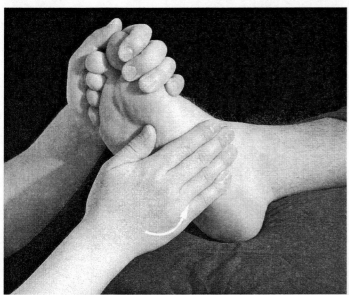

Circular stroking on the arch of the foot:

7 Stabilize the foot with your outer hand as in step 5. Place the palm of the inner hand in the middle of the arch. Use your fingertips as a pivot to maintain firm contact with the top of the arch. Remain in the same area during the entire stroke. Begin stroking up the inside of the foot with the palm of your hand. Use plenty of lubrication.

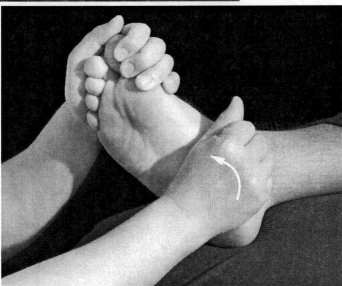

8 Continue the stroke on the arch with your palm. Begin making a circle by stroking toward the toes. Make sure the rotation is coming from your elbow and shoulder to minimize stress to your wrist.

9 Finish the stroke by circling in and down the arch back to the starting point. The circles should be large enough to cover the entire arch without having to move your fingertips. The size of the circles must be adjusted for each foot. Repeat 10 - 15 times. Again, you can combine straight and circular stroking techniques to smoothly cover the entire arch of the foot.

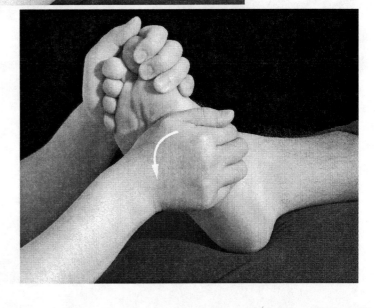

Japanese Foot Massage Techniques - Example #4

Vibrating the Feet

Japanese name of this technique

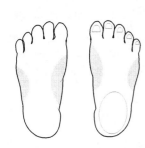

手掌 振せん法

Shu Ko Shin Sen Ho

The purpose of this technique

Relax the foot, ankle, leg, and knee

Where it is applied

On both (medial and lateral) edges of the feet

About this technique

This vibration technique is unique to Japanese foot massage. Vibration is used to shake the feet, ankles, and legs. It is a very important part of the warm up, but is often used in between other techniques to relax tension after the application of deep, stimulating techniques.

The technique consists of quickly flipping the foot back and forth between your hands. Start by practicing slowly. With practice and experience you will be able to perform it faster but you must learn to apply the technique properly first. When properly applied, the entire leg--from the foot to the upper thigh--should shake smoothly.

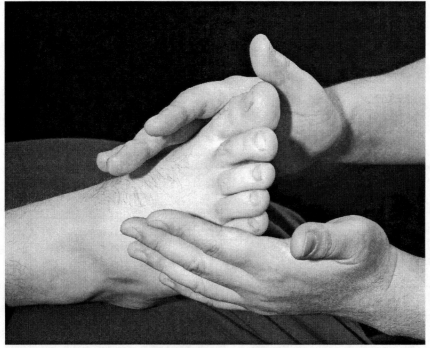

1 Begin by placing your hands on either side (medial and lateral sides) of the foot. Contact the sides of the foot with your palms at the base of the fingers. This is the neutral position. In this position, only the palms at the base of the fingers should be in contact with the foot.

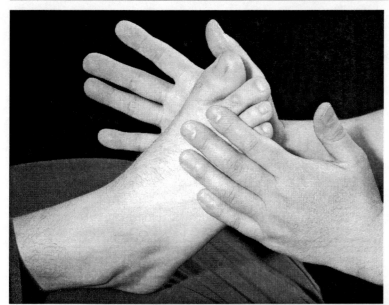

2 Gently rotate the inner (medial) edge of the foot away from you until the ball of the foot lays against your inner (right) palm. When the motion is complete, the fingers of your outer (left) hand should lay on the top (dorsal) of the foot with the foot resting between both hands. The fingers should not bend during this movement.

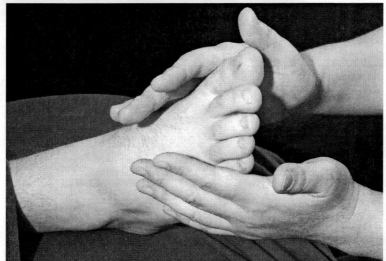

3 Return to the neutral position by rolling the inner edge of the foot back toward you. Continue by rotating the outer (lateral) edge of the foot away from you.

4 Rotate the foot until the ball of the foot lays against your outer palm, and the fingers of the inner hand lay on the top of the foot. This should be opposite of the positions in step 2.

5 Pivot your fingers back to the neutral position. Cycle ten times by going through steps 2, 3, 4, 3, and 2. Begin to slowly increase the speed until there is no pause in the neutral position.

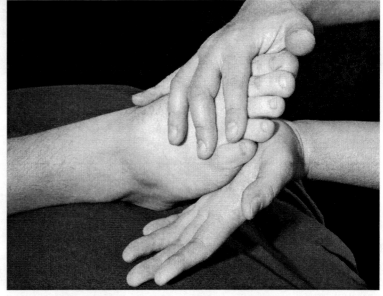

Japanese Foot Massage Techniques - Example #5

Stroking the Arches

Japanese name of this technique

把握軽擦法

Ha Aku Kei Satsu Ho

The purpose of this technique

Increase circulation and reduce muscle tension on the arch

Where it is applied

On the arches (along the medial longitudinal arch)

About this technique

This is one of the most fundamental techniques in Japanese foot massage, so practice until you are able to apply it smoothly. With practice, you should be able to increase the speed of your stroking until the client feels one continuous smooth stimulation. As you stroke faster, always make sure to start and end at the same place. Use enough lubrication so that you do not pull the client's skin.

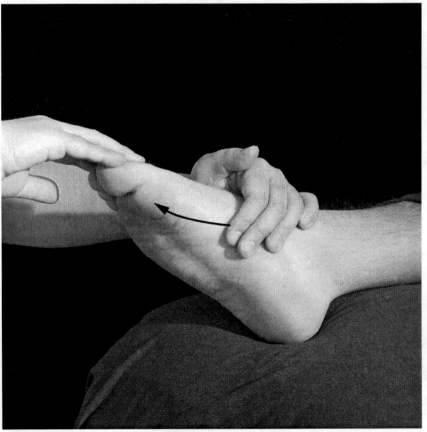

1 Grasp and gently squeeze the ankle between the palm and fingers of your outer (left) hand. Place the inner (right) hand gently on the top of the toes to stabilize the foot. Slide the outer hand up towards the big toe while continuing to squeeze. The pressure between the palm and the inside of your fingers should remain even. Do not apply too much pressure.

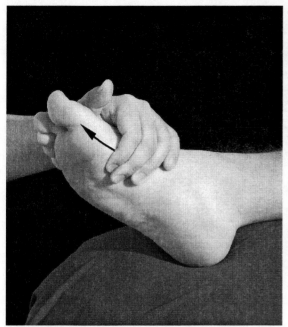

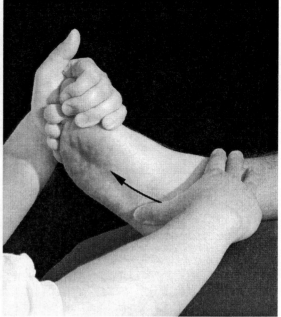

2 Remove the inner hand from the toes, while the outer hand continues the stroke up to the big toe.

3 As your outer hand approaches the big toe, place the inner hand over the ankle. Grasp and gently squeeze the ankle, applying even pressure between the palm and fingers of your inner hand.

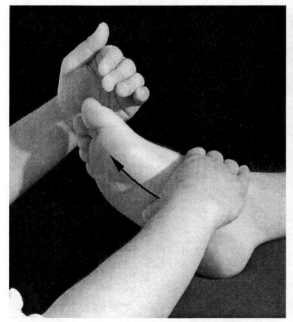

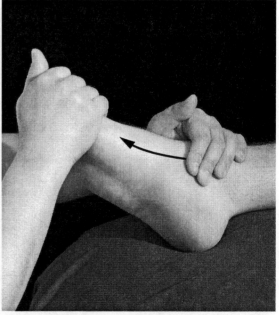

4 Remove your outer hand from the toes. Continue stroking up the arch toward the big toe with your inner hand. Again, apply even pressure between the palm and the inside of your fingers.

5 As you slide toward the toes with your inner hand, place the outer hand on the ankle and begin the sequence again. Repeat for 15 - 30 seconds. Concentrate on making the motion smooth, especially during the exchanges.

Japanese Foot Massage Techniques - Example #6

Thumb Stroking Over the Balls of the Feet

Japanese name of this technique

母指軽擦法

Bo Shi Kei Satsu Ho

The purpose of this technique

Reduce muscle tension over the ball of the foot

Where it is applied

Over the balls of the feet

About this technique

This technique strokes the ball of the foot with alternating thumbs and is performed rapidly with relatively light pressure. If you are applying slightly heavier pressure, slow down the rate of application to about one stroke per second. **Make sure that the foot itself is moving from left to right while applying this technique to avoid tiring your thumbs.** Use just enough lubrication to allow your thumbs to smoothly glide over the surface of the skin. More will be necessary for rapid strokes.

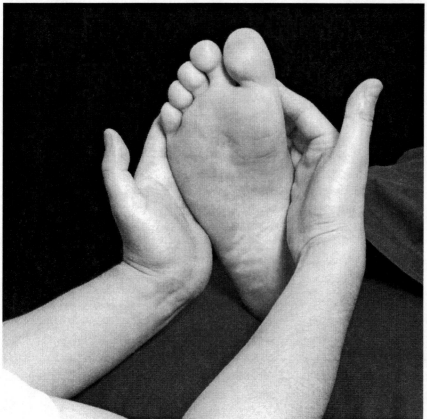

1 Place the foot between your hands and wrap your fingers over the top (dorsal) of the foot.

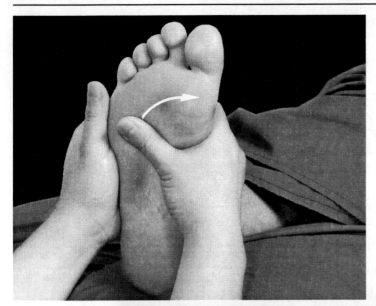

2 Place the tip of your inner (right) thumb beneath the smallest two toes just below the ball of the foot. Stroke quickly with light pressure over the ball of the foot until you reach the ball of the big toe. Make sure that you stroke with the entire side of the thumb, and not just with the tip.

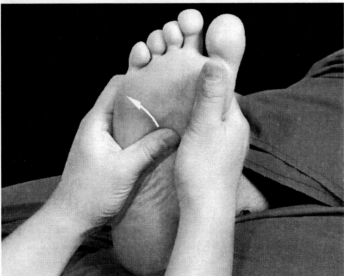

3 As you finish the stroke with the inner thumb, stroke with your outer (left) thumb from just below the ball of foot under the big toe, stroking up to the ball of the foot at the smallest (5th) toe.

4 As the outer thumb finishes its stroke, repeat again with the inner thumb. Keep your strokes even, light, and quick. Cover the entire ball of the foot. Practice until you are able to apply this smoothly. Applications should last between 10 - 15 seconds. Repeat stroking on the other foot.

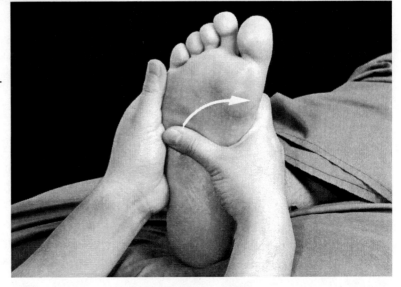

Japanese Foot Massage Techniques - Example #7

Thumb Stroking Up the Toes

Japanese name of this technique

母指軽擦法

Bo Shi Kei Satsu Ho

The purpose of this technique

To relax and improve the circulation of the toes

Where it is applied

On the bottom (plantar) side of the toes

About this technique

This example can be applied together with the previous example to warm the upper half of the foot and the toes. It can also be performed separately. Toes are very important for good structure of the body. They are also important for proper Ki flow in the body because the meridians begin and end at the toes.

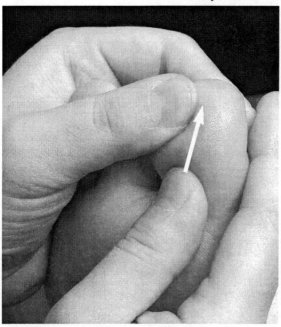
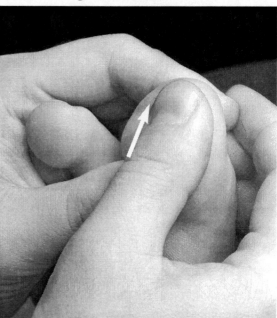

Straight up stroking on the big toe:

1 Place both hands around the foot so that the fingertips meet behind the toe for support while stroking. Place one thumb at the base of the big toe and the other thumb at the top of the big toe. Stroke with medium pressure from the base of the toe to the top.

2 As you finish the stroke with one thumb, alternate with the other thumb by bringing it to the base of the toe as the first one finishes its stroke. Strokes should be straight up. It is easy for the thumb to slip off of the toe when using lubricant, so be sure to stroke slowly.

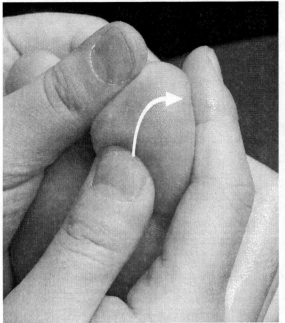 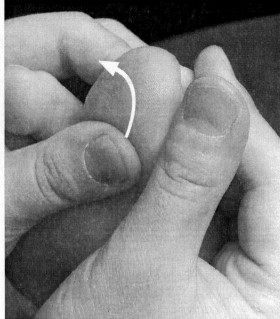

Curved up stroking on the big toe:

3 Use the same finger placement as in step 1. Start up-stroking with heavier pressure against the fingers. The big toe will automatically slide inward to make the curved stroke.

4 With the up-stroke of the other thumb, the big toe will automatically slide outward to make the curved stroke. Repeat for 4 - 6 strokes by alternating with both thumbs.

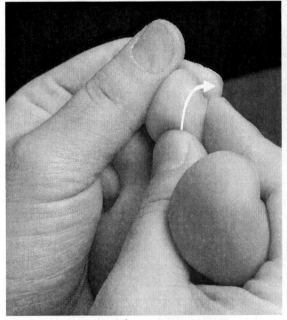 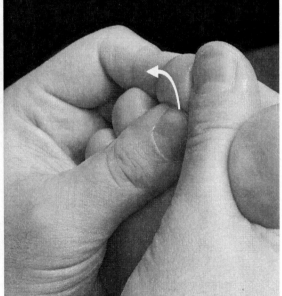

Curved up stroking on the small toes:

5 This is the same as steps 3 and 4, except it is applied on the other toes. Stroke 4 - 6 times with alternating thumbs as you move down to work on each toe.

6 Ease the pressure on the smaller toes. The fingers must be behind each toe for firm support so that the toe will not bend backward with the stroke.

Japanese Foot Massage Techniques - Example #8

Thumb Stroking Across the Middle of the Feet

Japanese name of this technique

母指軽擦法

Bo Shi Kei Satsu Ho

The purpose of this technique

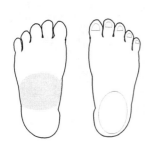

Increase circulation and reduce muscle tension on the middle of the sole

Where it is applied

Middle of the feet, in between the heels and the balls of feet

About this technique

This technique is excellent for warming and relaxing the foot in preparation for deeper work. It is very similar to Example #6 (Bo Shi Kei Satsu Ho), except that it is applied to the center of the foot instead of over the ball of the foot. As in Example #6, make sure that the foot is kept moving from left to right. The foot will not move as much in this example.

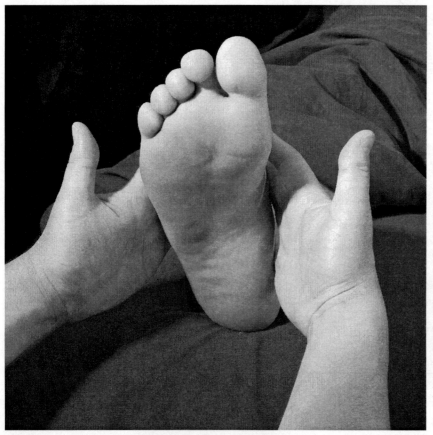

1 This is the same starting hand position as Example #6 except that the fingers of both hands are farther down toward the ankle. The fingertips should be touching each other on top (dorsal) of the foot with the pinkies of both hands touching the base of the leg where it meets the foot.

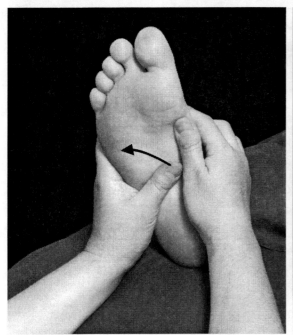

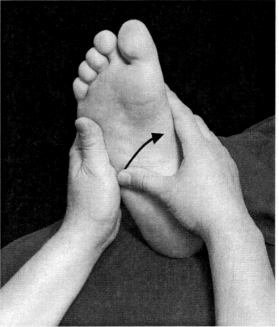

2 Place your outer (left) thumb across the foot just above the heel pad. Using light to medium pressure, stroke toward the smallest toe with the outer thumb. Be sure to stroke by using the entire side of the thumb, not just the tip.

3 Place your inner (right) thumb across the foot just above the heel pad. Stroke towards the big toe with the inner thumb. Alternate strokes with your thumbs and begin to move slowly down toward the heel.

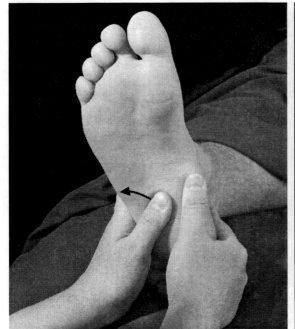

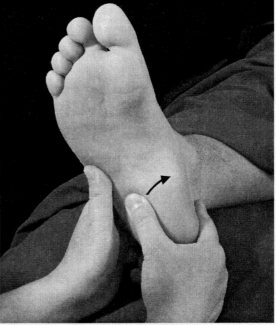

4 As you slide the hands downward across the ankle, toward the heel, the supporting fingers on the top of the foot must separate at the fingertips to maintain support.

5 As you reach the edge of the heel pad, make smaller strokes. Use just enough curvature to follow the contour of the heel pad. Work for about 10 - 20 seconds or until the foot is thoroughly warmed.

Japanese Foot Massage Techniques - Example #9

Thumb Stroking Up the Middle of the Feet

Japanese name of this technique

母指軽擦法

Bo Shi Kei Satsu Ho

The purpose of this technique

Reduce the muscle tension on the middle of the sole

Where it is applied

In the middle of the feet, in between the heels and balls of feet

About this technique

This technique often combines with the previous technique to gently stimulate the middle of the foot with the tips and upper parts of the thumbs. The movements in this technique come primarily from the shoulder and wrist, and not from the thumb. It can be used to stimulate the middle of the foot deeply, but the angle of the thumb must be raised to apply deeper pressure while the fingertips are hooked firmly around the top of the foot.

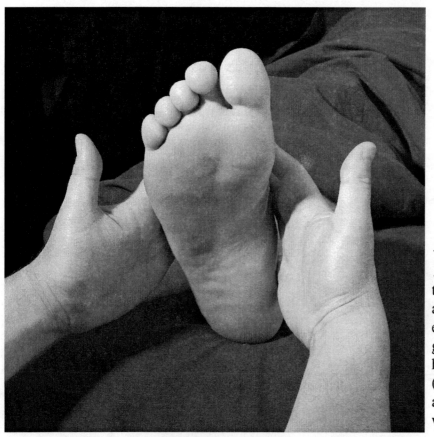

1 The placement of the hands in this technique is the same as the previous one, except less of the fingertips are used to hook around the top (dorsal) of the foot, and the angle of the wrist is higher.

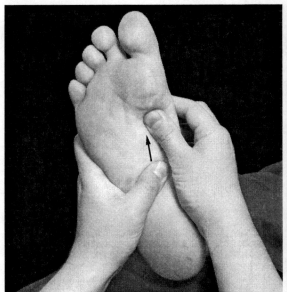

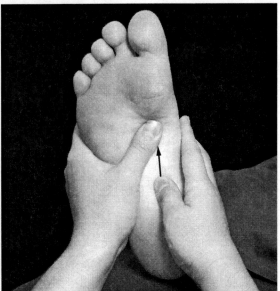

2 Place the inner (right) thumb just below the ball of the foot under the big toe for support. Place the tip of the outer (left) thumb just above the heel pad, next to the base of the arch. Stroke upward with the outer thumb toward the big toe. **Keep the thumb pointed upward to minimize stress to the thumb joint.**

3 As the outer thumb reaches just below the ball of the foot under the big toe, place the inner thumb where the left one started its stroke. Repeat the stroke with the inner thumb up to the ball of the foot. Stroke with alternating thumbs for 10 - 20 strokes.

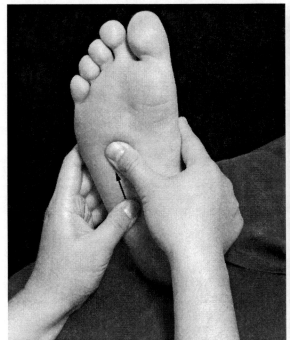

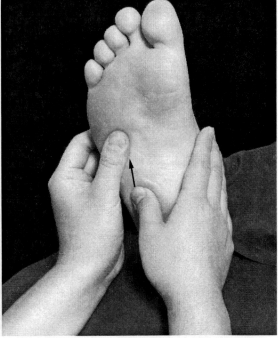

4 Move the thumbs one thumb-width at a time away from the arch. Repeat stroking in the middle of the foot with alternating thumbs as you did in steps 2 and 3.

5 Continue to move the thumbs one thumb-width at a time, repeating the strokes with alternating thumbs until just before the outside (lateral) edge of the foot.

Stroking the Arches with the Back of the Hand

Japanese name of this technique

指髁軽擦法

Shi Ka Kei Satsu Ho

The purpose of this technique

Improve circulation and reduce muscle tension of the arch

Where it is applied

On the arches and the surrounding regions of the feet

About this technique

This is a good example for releasing tension in the arch of the foot, especially if a client's feet fatigue easily. This example is applied with the back of the hand and fingers. **Do not stroke by using the knuckles of your closed fist.** This gives too strong of a stimulation because the angles of the knuckles are sharper. This is often uncomfortable for the client during the warm up. Keep your shoulders, elbows and wrists loose while applying this technique.

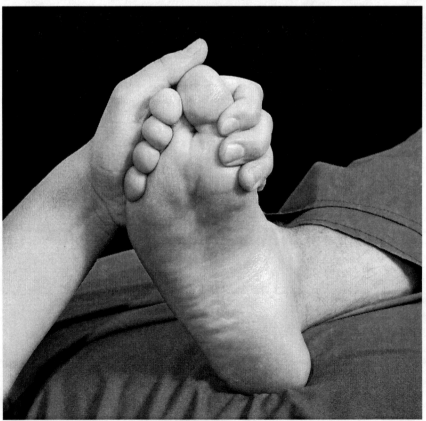

1 Grasp around toes of the foot with your outer (left) hand. Gently rotate the foot until the arch is exposed.

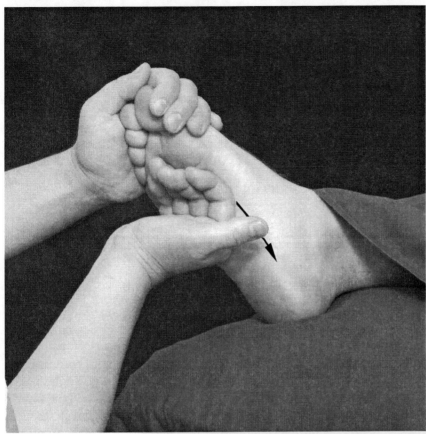

2 Fold the fingers of your inner (right) hand toward the palm and position the backs of your fingers and knuckles just below the ball of the foot under the big toe.

3 Apply firm pressure into the arch for support, then begin the stroke by gently pulling down with the outer hand on the toes. Stroke lightly along the arch, letting the inner hand close a bit further as you go downward. Maintain a fair amount of lubrication throughout the stroke.

4 Stop stroking just before the heel. Return the inner hand just under the ball of the foot, gently stroking upward, while releasing the foot with the outer hand. The fingers of the inner hand should open as you stroke back toward the toes.

5 Stroke back and forth, covering the entire arch. Repeat 10 - 15 times or as you desire.

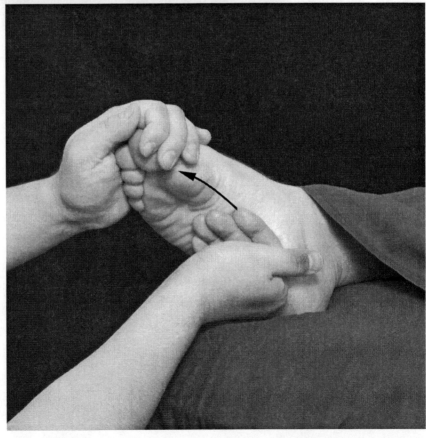

Japanese Foot Massage Techniques - Example #11

Rotation on the Arches with the Back of the Hand

Japanese name of this technique

指髁軽擦法

Shi Ka Kei Satsu Ho

The purpose of this technique

Improve circulation and reduce muscle tension of the arch

Where it is applied

On the arches of the feet

About this technique

This technique is very similar to the previous one and is often used in combination with it to reduce muscle tension on the middle of the arch. It is performed by using the backs of the fingers and hand, with the fingers folded over the palm (as was used in Example #10). **Again, do not use the knuckles of your closed fist during the warm up.** Make sure that rotations come from the elbow and shoulder and not from the wrist, although the wrist must be adjusted slightly to fit the contour of the arch.

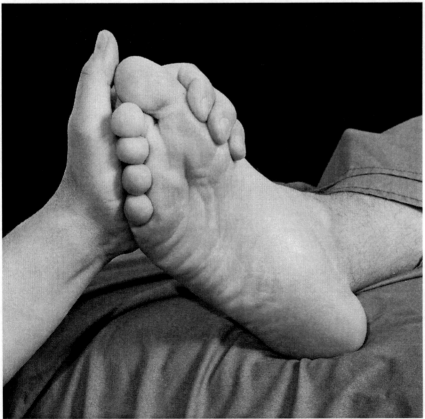

1 Hold the foot with your outer (left) hand the same way as you did in the previous example. Rotate the foot slightly further than in the previous example to better expose the arch.

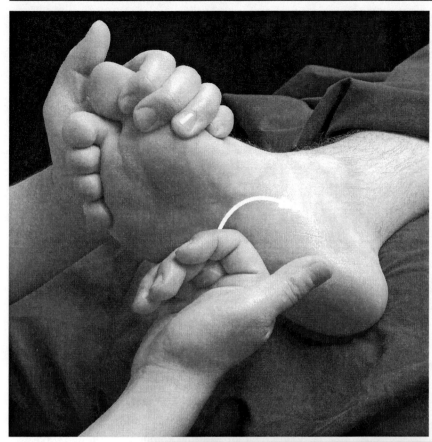

2 Fold the fingers of your inner (right) hand down over the palm so the tips are an inch or two away from the palm. Place the top (dorsal) surface of your fingers loosely in the arch. Rotate from elbow, not from the wrist, using plenty of lubrication. Make sure to keep the wrist, hand and fingers of the inner hand fairly firm.

3 Circular strokes should be large enough to cover the entire arch region from the ball of the foot below the big toe to the upper edge of the heel pad. If you like, you can gradually increase pressure while decreasing the speed of application as in the previous example. Apply this technique for 15 - 30 seconds, then repeat on the other foot.

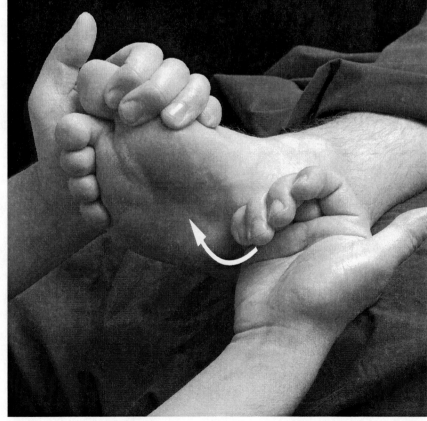

Japanese Foot Massage Techniques - Example #12

Combination Stroking in the Arches

Japanese name of this technique

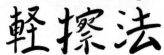

Kei Satsu Ho

The purpose of this technique

Reduce tension of the muscles and tendons of the arch

Where it is applied

On the arches and surrounding regions of the feet

About this technique

This technique is unique to Japanese foot massage. It is not the easiest technique to master, but it has great effects. In this example you will stroke the arch of the foot three times in each direction. It uses both sides (thenar and hypothenar - see p. 67) and the knuckles of the hand. If you move smoothly with faster speed, it will feel like one continuous stroke instead of three individual strokes. Practice is the key; it is best to give foot massages regularly and develop your technique over time. Good lubrication is necessary to apply this technique smoothly.

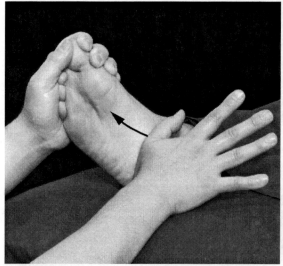

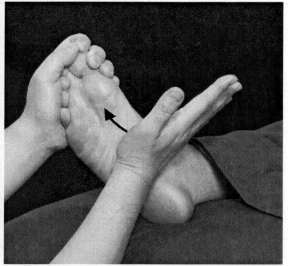

1 Grasp the top (dorsal) of the foot with your outer (left) hand. Gently rotate the foot so that the arch is exposed. Place the ball of the thumb (thenar side) of your inner (right) hand just above the heel pad. Stroke up along the arch with the thenar side of the hand towards the big toe with firm, even pressure.

2 As thenar side of the hand reaches just below the ball of the foot under the big toe, place the outside edge (hypothenar side) of the hand just above the heel pad, simultaneously removing the thenar side from the foot by turning the wrist. The outside edge of the hand then starts stroking up toward the big toe.

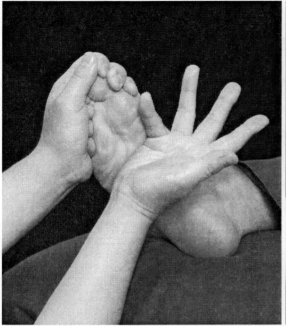

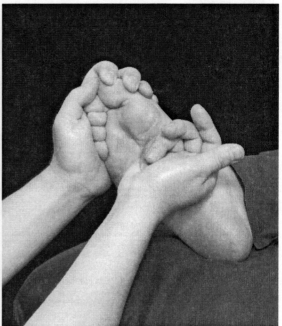

3 As you stroke toward the toes, continue rotating your wrist. Your palm should be facing upward, the fingers spreading as you stroke. Apply firm, even pressure with the outside edge of your hand while stroking.

4 Begin curling your fingers into your palm, one at a time, stopping just below the ball of the foot beneath the big toe.

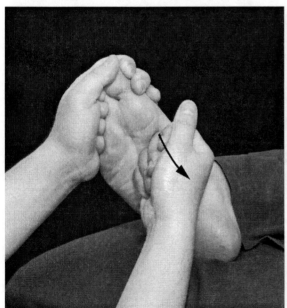

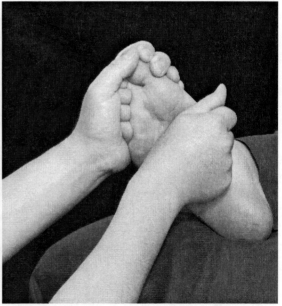

5 Finish closing your hand into a light fist and rotate your wrist so that the contact moves from the side of your hand to the back of the hand. Stroke downward along the arch with your knuckles by rotating the forearm.

6 You should stop the stroke when the rotation is complete and the thenar side of the hand is contacting the foot just above the heel pad. Then you can straighten the fingers and go back to starting position. Repeat the cycle 7 - 10 times.

Japanese Foot Massage Techniques - Example #13

Stroking Both Sides of the Achilles Tendons

Japanese name of this technique

四指軽擦法

Shi Shi Kei Satsu Ho

The purpose of this technique

Increase the circulation around the achilles tendon and the back of the ankle

Where it is applied

Both sides of the achilles tendons and the backs of the ankles

About this technique

This example can be combined with Example #14. As you stroke one side of the achilles tendon, simply continue the stroke down to the heel. You can then repeat this technique for the other side of the achilles tendon and heel. This technique requires a fair amount of lubrication, and it may require even more for someone with hairy legs.

During application of this technique it might be easier if you move your foot support slightly toward your client's head to create a space beneath the achilles tendons.

It is very beneficial to massage around the ankle so that proper Ki flow can be maintained. It is especially important to keep good Ki flow on the inside of the lower leg, on the side of the achilles tendon, and on the inner (medial) side of the ankle. This is where the three Yin Meridians are located on the legs (kidney, spleen and liver - see pp. 12 - 18).

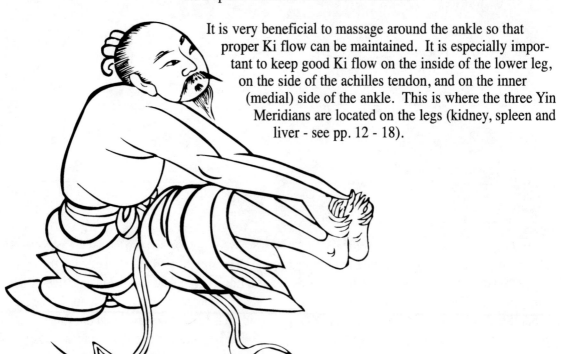

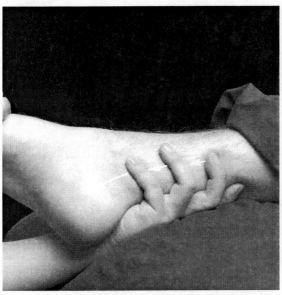 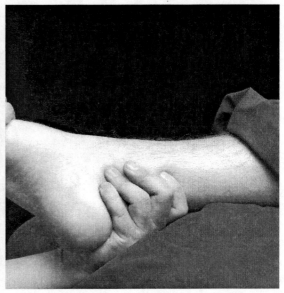

Inside (medial side) of the ankle:

1 Lightly place the inner (right) hand over the toes. Fan out the fingers of your outer (left) hand and place them under the top of the achilles tendon so that you can squeeze it between the fingers and palm.

2 Stroke down the side of the achilles tendon toward the heel. Apply firm pressure with the flats of your fingers as you compress them together. Stop at the heel (or continue into Example #14) and repeat several times.

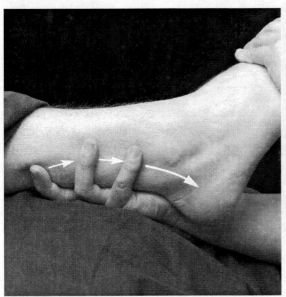 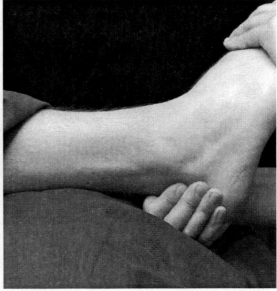

Outside (lateral side) of the ankle:

3 This is the same as the previous variation except that it is applied on the other side of the achilles tendon. Place your inner hand under the sides of the achilles tendons with the fingers fanned out.

4 Stroke toward yourself with firm pressure. As you stroke, pull separately with each of your fingers, and gather them together at the heel (or continue into Example #14). Repeat several times on each foot.

Japanese Foot Massage Techniques - Example #14

Finger Stroking Around the Heels

Japanese name of this technique

四指軽擦法

Shi Shi Kei Satsu Ho

The purpose of this technique

Reduce tension around the heel of the foot

Where it is applied

Behind the ankles and backs of the heels

About this technique

This technique is generally combined with the previous one. Stroke down the achilles tendon to the ankle and spread your fingers as you pass over it. Even when combined, you will actually be making two separate strokes.

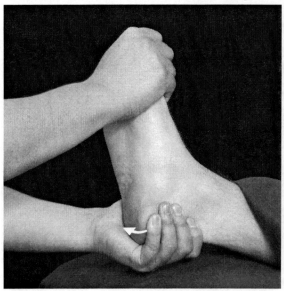

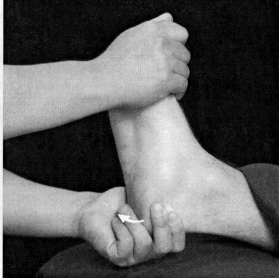

Inside (medial side) of the heel:

1 Grasp the top (dorsal) of the foot around the toes with your inner (right) hand. Grasping the heel with the palm of the outer (left) hand, place the fingers behind the heel so that the index finger is touching the achilles tendon. Place the base of the thumb on the other side of the heel for firm support. Start stroking the side of the heel with the pinky using firm pressure. It will naturally slide off from the heel.

2 Keeping the stroke smooth, continue by letting each finger slide off from the heel. Maintain firm pressure with the fingers while each finger follows the previous one in a fanning movement around the heel ending with the index finger. Make sure that each finger is stroking separately around the heel, instead of all the fingers at the same time. Repeat 3 - 5 times.

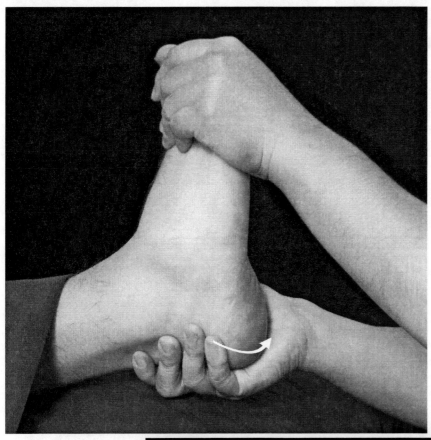

Outside (lateral side) of the heel:

This variation is applied with the inner hand on the outside of the heel.

3 For this variation, grasp the top of the foot with the outer (left) hand. Place the inner hand under the heel, starting the stroke with the pinky finger in the same way as applied in step 1.

4 Continue by letting each finger slide off from the heel. Each finger must maintain firm pressure, so that as it reaches the end of the heel, it falls off firmly into your palm.

5 Repeat 3 - 5 times, concentrating on making the stroke smooth and even. Repeat both procedures on the other foot.

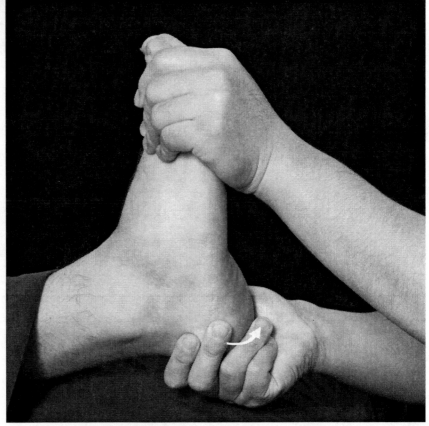

Light Stroking Down with Both Hands

Japanese name of this technique

把握軽擦法

Ha Aku Kei Satsu Ho

The purpose of this technique

Relax the foot and give a smooth finish to the entire massage

Where it is applied

On the tops and bottoms (dorsas and plantars) of the feet

About this technique

This is the final example of the warm up techniques, and is applied gently and slowly. It is also often used as a nice, smooth way to finish the entire massage. This example shows two different variations of stroking. Generally, one variation is sufficient for this technique, and you may choose the one that is most comfortable for you. Use a fair amount of lubrication.

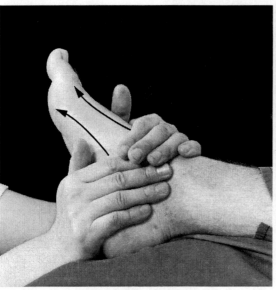
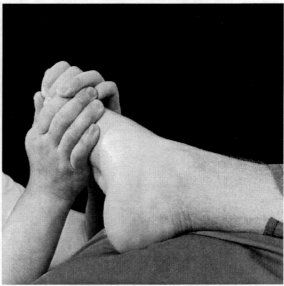

Top and bottom of the foot:

1 Grasp the foot between your palms and the fingers of both hands, one hand placed on the top (dorsal) of the foot and the other under the heel, slightly overlapping the fingers by the ankle. Start stroking by pulling both slowly hands toward the toes with firm, even pressure.

2 Continue stroking toward the toes until you reach the base of the big toe. Repeat this technique several times as you desire.

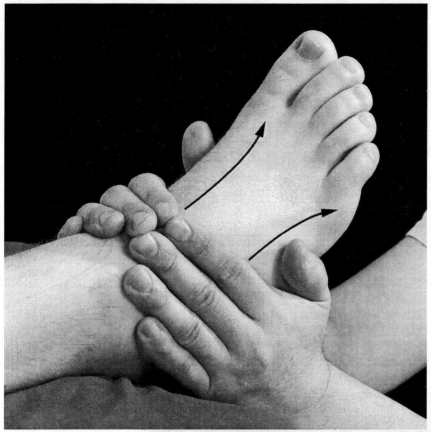

Sides of the foot:

3 This is very similar to the previous variation, except that the palms should be placed on either side of the foot. The fingers contact each other at the top of the foot with the palms covering each ankle.

4 Start stroking with firm pressure by slowly pulling both hands toward the toes. Try to keep as much of the hands and fingers in contact with the foot as possible. Make sure to use plenty of lubrication.

5 Stop stroking when you reach the toes. Repeat several times as desired.

When you complete all of the warm up techniques on one foot, return to Example #1 on page 98 and repeat all of the warm up techniques on the other foot.

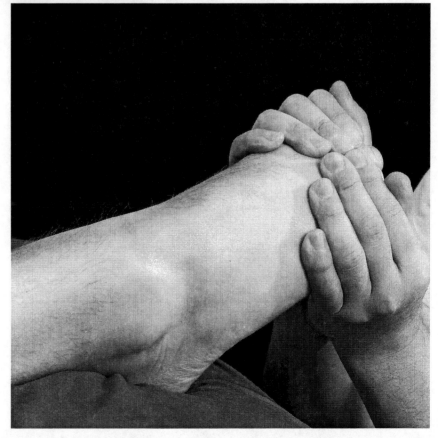

Chapter Eight

JAPANESE FOOT MASSAGE TECHNIQUES

With Lubrication

In the previous chapter, I introduced light, smooth warm up techniques. In this chapter, I will introduce fifteen deep-stimulating techniques of Japanese foot massage that are for working at a therapeutic level. These techniques are also performed in the supine position with lubrication.

While the warm up techniques are generally performed as a group to warm up the entire foot, the techniques shown in this chapter should be selected based on the particular condition or region of the foot and used as needed.

In this chapter, I will provide examples of several techniques in specific regions of the foot. For example, the first five examples of techniques in this chapter work specifically on the balls of the feet. After practicing techniques for a specific area, you should try to combine them with the warm up techniques to create your own method of therapeutic foot massage. Later, you can combine them with the stretching techniques found in Chapter 10.

When you perform these examples, the supporting hand is as important as the applying hand (if not more important). In Japanese foot massage you can apply the techniques in any order as long as you begin by applying lighter pressure and gradually increase it. Make sure to adjust the amount of pressure you use to the client's sensitivity. If you use greater pressure, apply the technique more slowly. It is best to go back and forth between different techniques to flow smoothly and reduce risk of over-stressing the hand muscles by using the same particular movement.

Alternate Thumb Stroking Between the Metatarsals

Japanese name of this technique

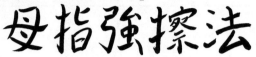

Bo Shi Kyo Satsu Ho

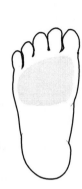

The purpose of this technique

Reduce muscle tension between the metatarsals

Where it is applied

Between the metatarsal on the soles of the feet

About this technique

The next five examples show how to deeply stimulate the ball of the foot. When applying this technique, use slow and smooth strokes. Avoid rapid strokes. **For this technique, your thumb should always be pointed toward the ceiling--not inward--so that it does not stress the thumb joints. Also, the thumb must be kept completely straight, do not bend it while stroking.** Make sure that the stroke is applied from shoulder and elbow movement, and not just from the thumb and wrist.

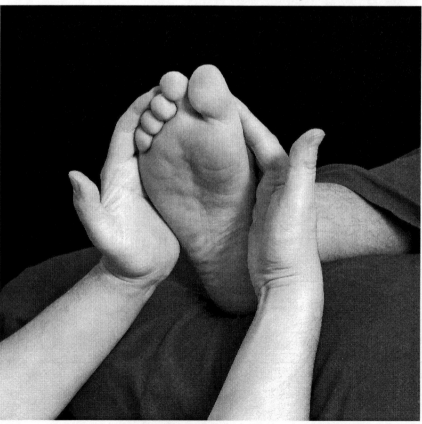

1 Apply a small amount of lubricant to your thumbs. Place the fingers of both hands on the top (dorsal) of the foot. The index fingers should meet over the big toe and the second toe.

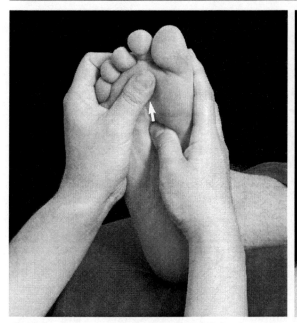

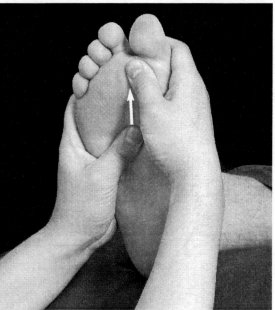

2 Place your thumbs on the ball of the foot in the hollow between the first two foot bones (metatarsals and phlangeals). Apply heavy pressure with the tip of the inner (right) thumb just below the ball of the foot. Stroke upward between the bones with the inner thumb.

3 Stroke up to the base of the toes. As the inner thumb reaches the top of the ball of the foot, place the outer (left) thumb at the starting point and repeat the stroke with the outer thumb. Alternate strokes in the hollow between the first two foot bones 4 - 10 times.

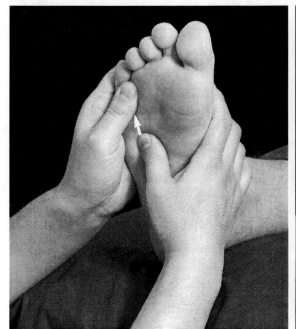

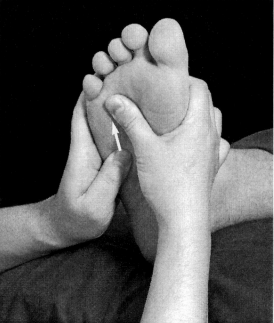

4 Separate the bones slightly as you stroke up between the bones of the foot to loosen the tissue. After several strokes move down to the next set of foot bones and repeat the stroking.

5 Continue moving down the foot until finishing between the fourth and fifth bones. Then repeat the stroking on the left foot.

Japanese Foot Massage Techniques - Example #17

Deep Thumb Stroking Between the Metatarsals

Japanese name of this technique

母指強擦法

Bo Shi Kyo Satsu Ho

The purpose of this technique

Reduce muscle tension on the ball of the foot

Where it is applied

Between the metatarsal bones on the balls of the feet

About this technique

This example is similar to the previous one, except that only one thumb is used to stroke and it is a much deeper technique. Make sure that you stroke by utilizing the movement of the outer (lateral) hand to bring the foot toward you, in order to minimize stress to the thumb.

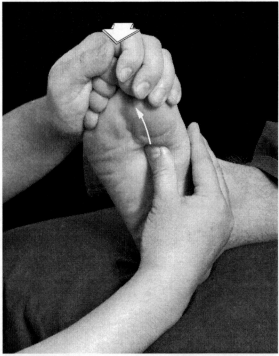

1 Grasp the foot over the toes with your outer (left) hand to stabilize it. Apply a small amount of lubricant. Place the tip of thumb of the inner (right) hand just below the ball of the foot under the big toe between the first and second foot bones (metatarsals).

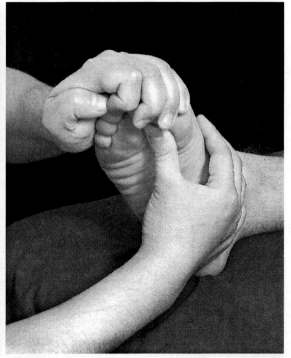

2 Stroke toward the toe by bringing the outer hand forward (toward you). Move the inner thumb slightly to adjust the angle to the foot, but do not stroke with the thumb. Stop stroking just before you reach the web between the toes.

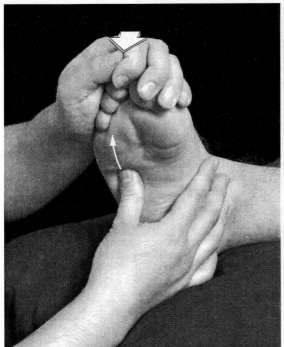

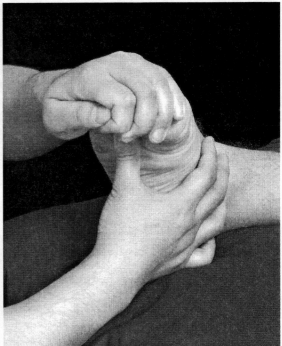

3 Move to the next set of foot bones, stroking 3 - 5 times for each set, always stopping just before the webbing between the toes.

4 Work until you have finished stroking between the fourth and fifth foot bones. Repeat on the other foot.

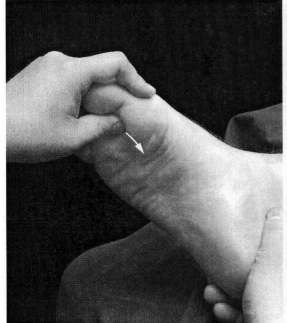

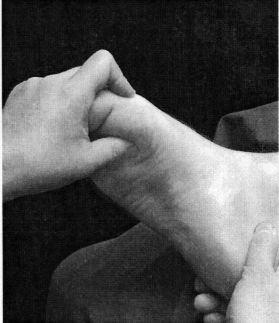

A lternatively, you can stroke with the thumb from the toes toward the heel, but this is generally not as easy to apply and is less effective. Grasp the heel with your inner hand and place the thumb of your outer hand at the base between two toes. Stroke from the base of each toe toward the heel. Stroke as far as the thumb will reach, although you may not be able to stroke as far as you did in steps 1 - 4. Again, begin work the hollows between the first and second foot bones and repeat through the fourth and fifth.

Cross Stroking Over the Balls of the Feet

Japanese name of this technique

母指強擦法

Bo Shi Kyo Satsu Ho

The purpose of this technique

Reduce the muscles tension on the balls of the foot

Where it is applied

On the balls and the upper outside (lateral) edges of the feet

About this technique

This and the two previous examples are good for loosening the muscles and tendons over the foot bones (metatarsals and phalangeals). Although the muscles and tendons of the foot are strong enough to support the weight of the entire body, firmly massaging this area can be helpful to reduce fatigue.

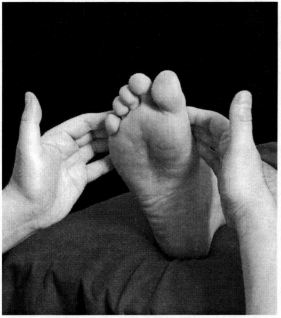

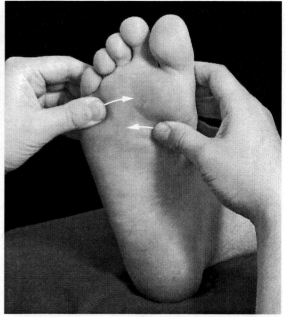

1 Place the fingers of both hands on the top (dorsal) of the foot for support. The fingertips of the inner (right) hand should lightly hook in the hollow between the first and second foot bones (metatarsals), and the fingers of your outer (left) hand should lightly hook between the fourth and fifth foot bones.

2 Place the inner thumb on the ball of the foot under the big toe (over the first metatarsal) and the outer thumb on the ball of the foot under the smallest toe (over the fifth metatarsal). Slide the thumbs toward each other using moderate pressure. Allow the foot to move slightly back away from you with the pressure of the stroke.

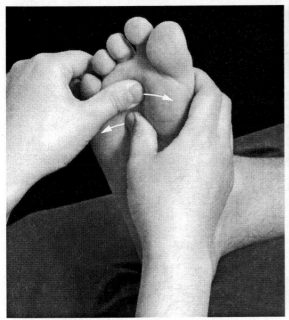

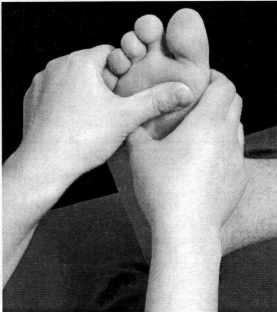

3 The thumbs should cross at the center of the ball of the foot. It is not important which goes above the other, use whichever is most comfortable. Continue to stroke toward the edges of the foot with lighter pressure to minimize movement of the supporting fingers.

4 Each thumb should finish the stroke at the edge of the ball of the foot. Move to stroke slightly above or below the ball of the foot, repeating this technique 10 - 15 times to cover the entire area.

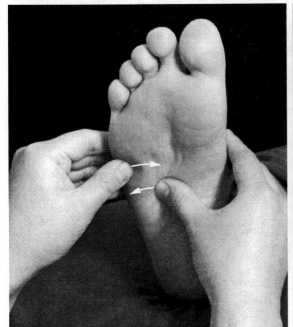

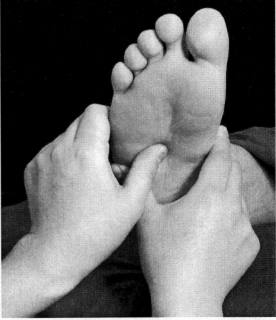

5 Using the same concept, continue stroking with smaller strokes as you move down the outside (lateral) edge of the foot, shifting the starting point of the inner thumb to the center of the middle of the foot.

6 After each stroke, move down one thumb width toward the heel and repeat until you reach the top of the heel pad. Repeat 2 - 3 times on the lateral edge of each foot's midsection.

Japanese Foot Massage Techniques - Example #19

Thumb Stroking Across the Base of the Toes

Japanese name of this technique

母指頭揉捏法

Bo Shi To Kyo Satsu Ho

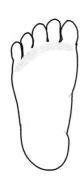

The purpose of this technique

Reduce tension on the muscles and tendons at the base of each toe

Where it is applied

At the base of each toe

About this technique

The previous example loosens most parts of the the balls of the feet. You will find that this technique works well at the base of each toe, although application is difficult in this area. To maximize the benefits of this technique use as much pressure as the client is comfortable with. Use only enough lubricant to allow your thumbs to slide over the skin smoothly--too much lubricant will prevent the application of deeper pressure. To apply with lighter pressure, use the softer, flatter part of your thumb. For heavier pressure, use just the tip of the thumb by the fingernail, without letting the fingernail touch the foot during application.

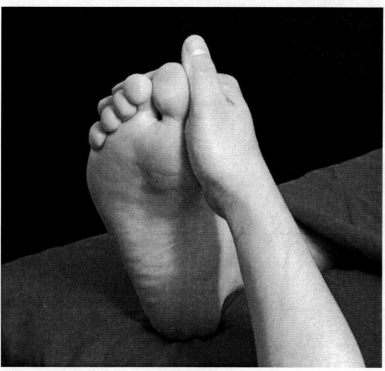

1 Cup the top (dorsal) of the foot with your inner (right) hand. The thumb should be next to the big toe and the heel of the hand should be on the side of the ball of the foot by the big toe. The rest of the hand should wrap around the top side of the foot. If the ankle is stiff, help to loosen by wiggling the foot from side to side several times. If it remains stiff, return to Examples #4 and #5 and apply them until the ankle releases its tension.

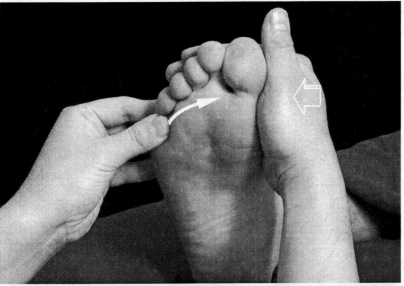

2 Place the thumb of the outer (left) hand between the ball of the foot under the smallest toe and the toe itself. It should be angled toward the palm of the inner (right) hand. Applying moderate or heavy pressure, slide the tip of the thumb slowly toward the base of the big toe by using the inner hand to gradually push the foot toward the outer thumb.

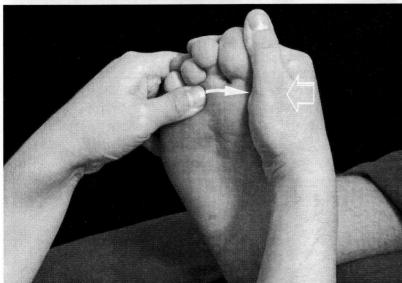

3 Continue slowly stroking the upper edge of the ball of the foot by pushing the inner hand toward the outer thumb as it slides over the base of one toe to the base of the next. Be sure to keep the outer thumb straight while pressure is being applied. The foot should be well supported with the inner hand.

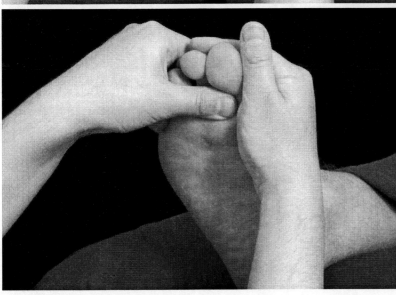

4 Finish the stroke at the base of the big toe. The tip of the outer thumb should meet the ball of the inner thumb. Repeat several times on each foot. Always begin with the little toe and work towards the big toe, with the outer thumb pointing toward the inner hand. If possible, increase pressure slightly with each repetition.

Japanese Foot Massage Techniques - Example #20

Deep Thumb Kneading Between the Metatarsals

Japanese name of this technique

母指頭揉捏法

Bo Shi To Ju Netsu Ho

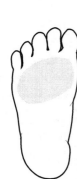

The purpose of this technique

Reduce muscle tension between the foot bones

Where it is applied

Between the foot bones (metatarsals and phalangeals) on the balls of the feet

About this technique

This technique uses the outside (lateral) edges of both thumbs to knead between the foot bones. A little lubrication is necessary, but too much will make it difficult to stroke deeply. Slow the kneading as you work deeper, but do not work so deeply that it is painful to the client. It is best to keep the pressure at the therapeutic level where they could experience slight discomfort, but they should not feel pain. It is essential to adjust the amount of pressure you apply to the sensitivity of the client.

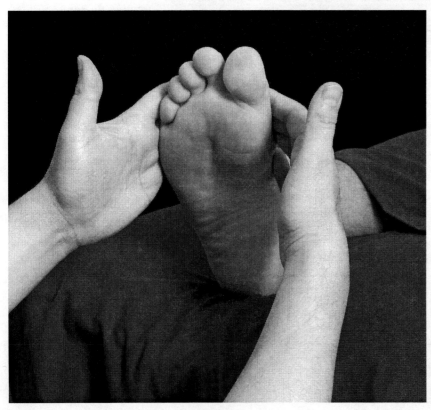

1 Place the fingers of both hands on the top (dorsal) of the foot. The fingers of the inner (right) hand should hook over the first foot bone (metatarsal) and the fingers of the outer (left) hand should hook over the fifth foot bone.

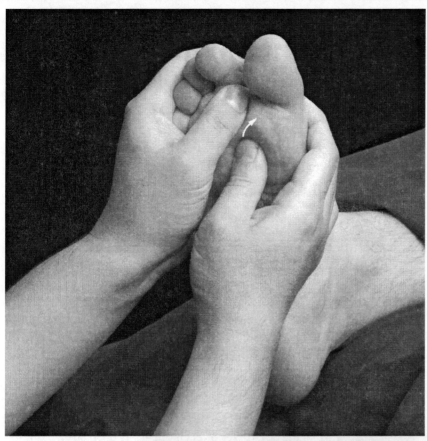

2 Place the thumbs between the first two foot bones so that the outer thumb is at the base of the second toe and the inner thumb is at the base of the ball of the foot under the big toe.

3 Lightly squeeze the foot between your hands. Apply short, curved strokes to the outer (lateral) edge of the first foot bone with the outside (lateral) tip of the inner thumb. Stroking should be applied with heavy pressure to loosen the muscles and slightly separate the bones.

4 As the inner thumb finishes its upward stroke, continue by repeating the stroke on the inner (medial) edge of the second foot bone with the outer thumb. Alternate the thumbs, one after another, to create a deep kneading stroke. With each stroke, the thumbs should move down little by little toward the heel, until just past the ball of the foot. Start at the top of the next set of foot bones, and repeat the kneading between all of the foot bones on both feet.

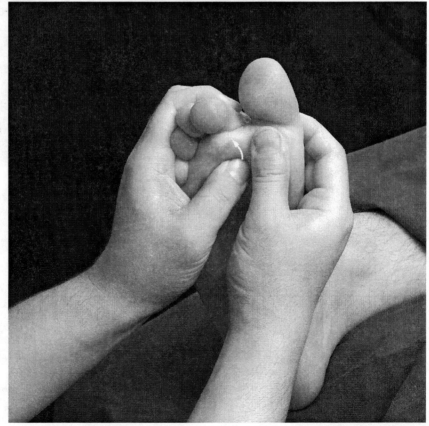

Japanese Foot Massage Techniques - Example #21

Deep Stroking on the Arches Using the Knuckles

Japanese name of this technique

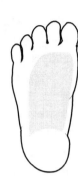

手拳強擦法

Shu Ken Kyo Satsu Ho

The purpose of this technique

Reduce muscle tension and help restore arches

Where it is applied

On the arches and surrounding regions of the feet

About this technique

The next five examples are applied to the arch of the foot. The Shu Ken Kyo Satsu Ho is similar to Example #10 (Shi Ka Kei Satsu Ho) except that it is applied with the knuckles of the fist instead of the backs of the fingers. This gives much deeper stimulation. Make sure that the foot has been adequately warmed with other techniques before applying a deep stimulating technique such as this one. If the feet are sensitive to pressure, adjust according to the sensitivity of each client. If deep stimulation is not required, this example may be omitted.

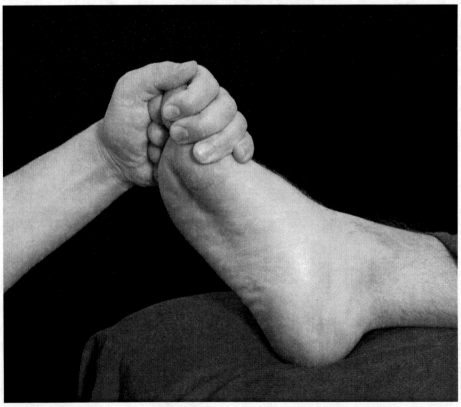

1 Grasp the toes of the foot with your outer (left) hand. Adjust for better access by slightly rotating the foot until the arch is exposed.

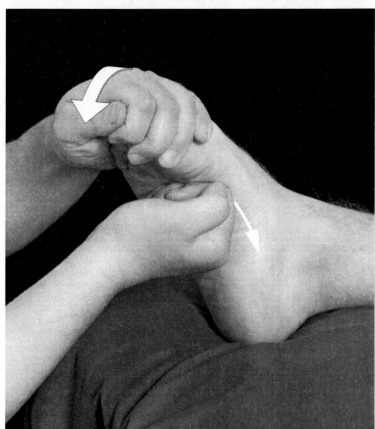

2 Place the knuckles of your closed inner (right) fist just below the ball of the foot under the big toe. Stroke down the arch toward the heel with the knuckles, while the outer (left) hand gently pushes down on the top of the foot. For a deeper stroke, use the fingers and palm on top of the foot, as shown below, to increase downward pressure (instead of pushing harder with the knuckles). Your inner wrist should be kept fairly stiff during the entire stroke.

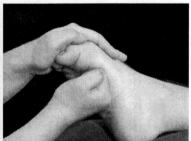

3 Stroke back toward the balls of the foot with the knuckles, while releasing pressure on the top of the foot. The pressure of the hands during the up stroke is not quite as strong as the down stroke, but the hands should remain in firm contact. Repeat five to ten times on each foot. With each repetition, continue to stroke slowly, while gradually increasing the pressure.

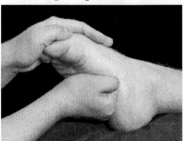

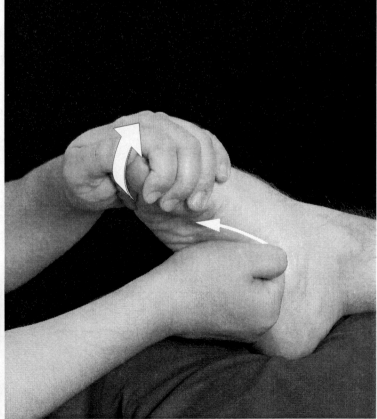

Japanese Foot Massage Techniques - Example #22

Circular Stroking on the Edges of the Arches

Japanese name of this technique

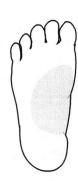

母指軽擦法

Bo Shi Kei Satsu Ho

The purpose of this technique

Reduce muscle tension and increase circulation on the arch

Where it is applied

On the edges of the arches of the feet

About this technique

This example applies circular stroking around the edge of the arch to give slightly deeper stimulation to the entire region. If you want to give even deeper stimulation, apply with more pressure or use the next examples. Keep the thumbs (carpometacarpal or metacarpophalangeal joints) locked, and rotate by moving the foot with your outer hand. **The majority of the rotation comes from the outer hand** (the one grasping the toes). There is little movement coming from the thumbs alone. **Do not try to stroke with the thumb.**

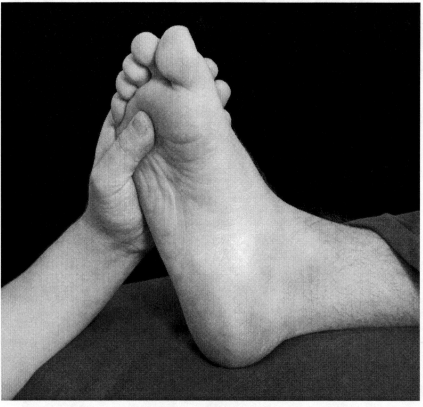

1 Grasp the top (dorsal) of the foot, slightly higher than midway with your outer (left) hand. The thumb should be across the ball of the foot and the fingers should be across the top of the foot.

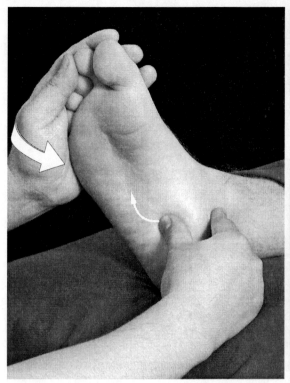

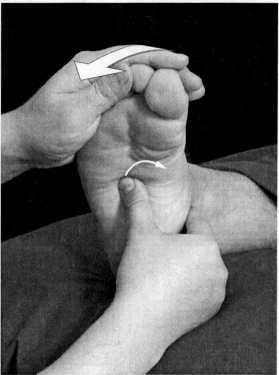

2 Place the tip of your inner (right) thumb at the edge of the arch, just above the heel. Push the foot inward and down into the thumb, so that the thumb strokes up toward the toes.

3 From there, stroke with the thumb until it reaches the inside (medial) edge by pulling the foot outward with the outer hand. You are moving the foot so the thumb will trace a large circle.

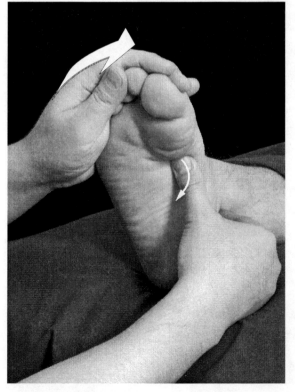

4 Finally, push the foot inward and up so the thumb strokes down the arch and back to the starting position to finish the circle. Maintain fairly strong, even pressure with your arm while keeping the thumb as stationary as possible. Repeat for 5 - 10 circular strokes.

Japanese Foot Massage Techniques - Example #23

Stroking the Middle of the Feet with the Thumb

Japanese name of this technique

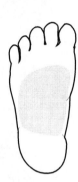

母指強擦法

Bo Shi Kyo Satsu Ho

The purpose of this technique

Reduce tension in the muscles and tendons in middle of the foot

Where it is applied

On the middle of the feet and surrounding regions

About this technique

This technique is similar to Example #9. However, this example is applied much deeper and slower at a therapeutic level than at a warming level. This technique is good for reducing tension between the foot bones (metatarsals) and stretching the tendons and muscles of the foot. This region can be very tight or sore on some people, especially those who spend long hours standing or walking. Work it carefully and thoroughly, adjusting pressure according to each client's level of sensitivity.

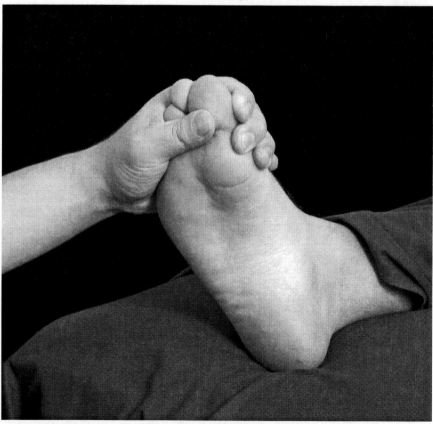

1 Grasp the toes and the top (dorsal) of the foot with your outer (left) hand.

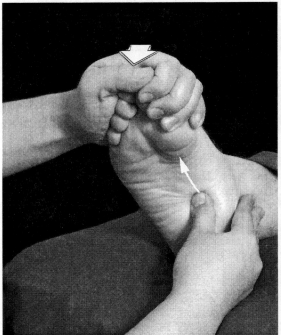

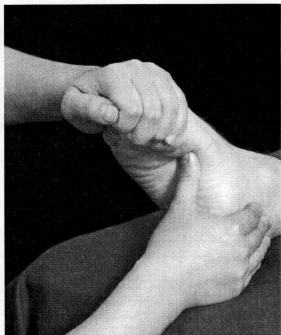

2 Place the thumb of the inner (right) hand just above the heel pad in the middle of the foot. Stroke up toward the ball of the foot under big toe by pulling the foot down into the inner thumb.

3 Stop stroking just below the ball of the foot under the big toe. Do not stroke with the thumb. Pull the foot into the thumb and adjust the angle of the thumb as needed, but do not hyperextend.

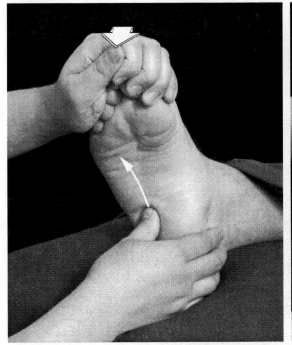

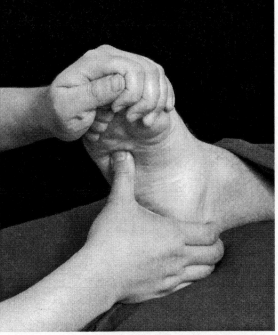

4 Return to the same starting hand positions as steps 1 - 3. This time, stroke upward on the outer (lateral) edge with the inner thumb by pulling the foot down toward yourself.

5 Finish the stroke just below the ball of the foot under the fifth toe. Repeat 3 - 5 times on each foot.

Japanese Foot Massage Techniques - Example #24

Circular Stroking on the Arches

Japanese names of these techniques

母指球軽擦法

Bo Shi Kyu Kei Satsu Ho (steps 1-2)
Ko Shi Kyu Kei Satsu Ho (steps 3-5)

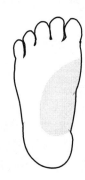

The purpose of these techniques

Reduce muscle tension on the arch and surrounding areas

Where they are applied

On the arches of the feet

About these techniques

This example applies small circular stroking on the arch to reduce muscle tension. There are two variations of this example. Choose the one that best fits the size of your hands, the size of the client's foot, and the rotation of the ankle. If you are applying with heavier pressure, use less lubricant. Stroking comes from the movement of the elbow and shoulder, not the wrist.

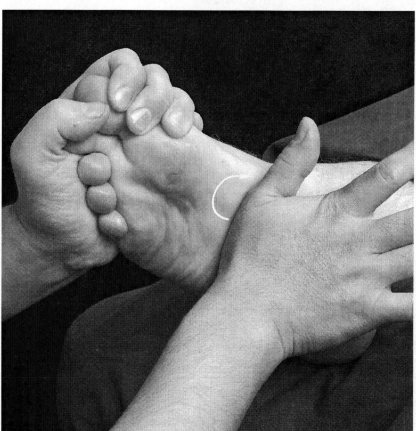

Base of the thumb:

1 Grasp the top (dorsal) of the foot and toes with your outer (left) hand.

2 Place the base of your thumb (thenar side) into the arch of the foot and stroke in a small, circular motion. These movements should be fairly rapid and move over the surface of the skin. Always stroke from your elbow and shoulder, not from the wrist. Cover the entire arch from just below the ball of the foot under the big toe to the top of the heel pad.

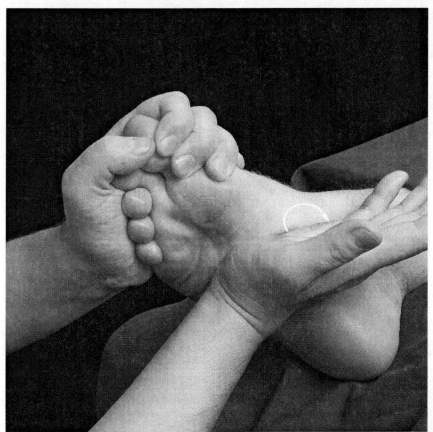

Base of the side of the hand:

3 This is similar to the previous variation, but it is applied by placing the pinky (hypothenar) side of the hand into the arch of the foot. Again, stabilize the foot with your outer hand. Use fairly rapid movements to stroke in small, circular motions.

4 Cover the entire arch region with the circular movements. Adjust the angle of your hands to the foot to best fit the contour of the arch. Repeat on the other foot.

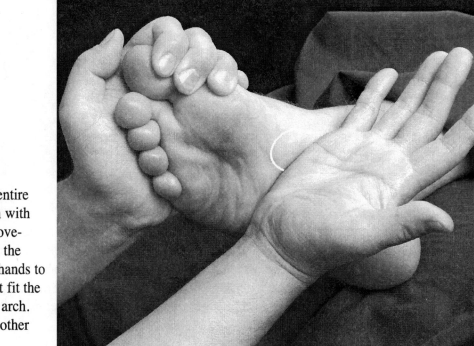

Japanese Foot Massage Techniques - Example #25

Stroking Inward Over the Arches

Japanese name of this technique

母指軽擦法

Bo Shi Kei Satsu Ho

The purpose of this technique

Reduce muscle tension and help restore the contour of the arch

Where it is applied

On the arches of the feet

About this technique

This example is designed for deep stimulation on the inside of the arch. Many people have tension and pain in the arch just above the heel pad. If the client experiences pain it indicates that extra work is required, so start the application gently, keeping your strokes slow as you gradually increase the amount of pressure. Continue working at the therapeutic level (which will cause slight discomfort). Use a fair amount of lubricant, but too much can make it difficult to apply deep pressure.

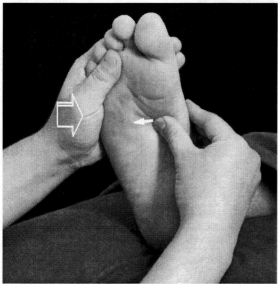

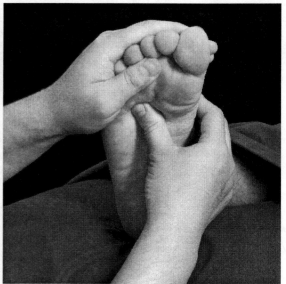

1 Grasp the top (dorsal) of the foot with the outer (left) hand, so the palm supports the outside (lateral) edge of the foot. Place the tip of the inner (right) thumb just below the ball of the foot under the big toe on the inside edge (medial edge of first metatarsal), pointing toward the outer hand.

2 Stroke by pushing the foot into the inner thumb with the outer hand instead of stroking with the thumb. Maintain medium to heavy pressure during the stroke, while the inner thumb slides over the arch, stopping at the center of the foot.

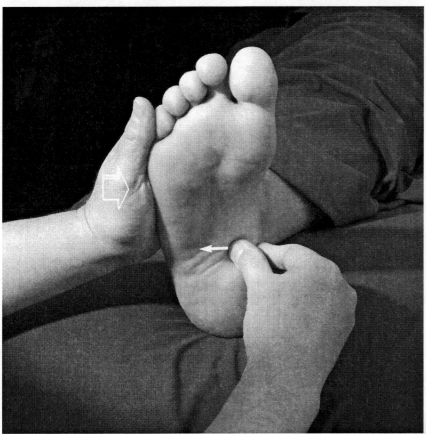

3 Move the inner thumb down one thumb-width and repeat. You should also move the outer hand down so that you can press the foot into the inner thumb. Continue moving down one thumb-width at a time, pressing the arch of the foot into the thumb. Continue until the thumb reaches the top of the heel pad.

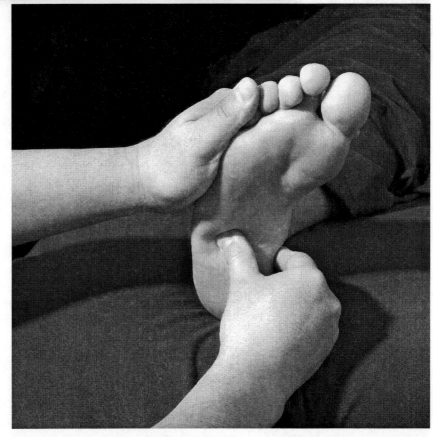

4 Repeat the entire sequence 2 - 3 times from top to bottom along the entire arch. Then repeat on the other foot.

Japanese Foot Massage Techniques - Example #26

Stroking Inward from the Edges of the Feet

Japanese name of this technique

母指頭強擦法

Bo Shi To Kyo Satsu Ho

The purpose of this technique

Reduce muscle tension on the outside (lateral) half of the foot

Where it is applied

On the outside (lateral) half of the balls and middle of the feet

About this technique

This example uses the same concept as the previous one, except that the stroking is applied to the outside (lateral) half of the foot and the stroking is toward the inside (medial) edge. It requires slight lubrication, but not so much that you cannot apply firm pressure. It is an excellent technique for people who have sore feet or for those who are on their feet for long periods of time.

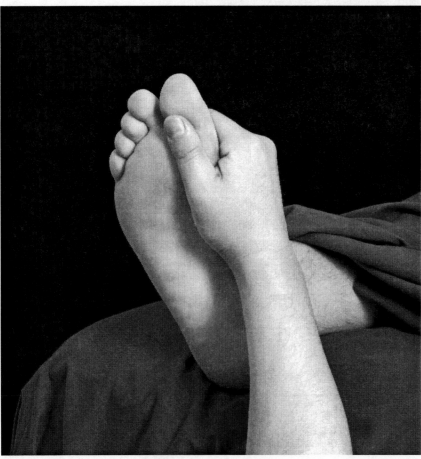

1 Grasp around the ball of the foot under the big toe with your inner (right) hand.

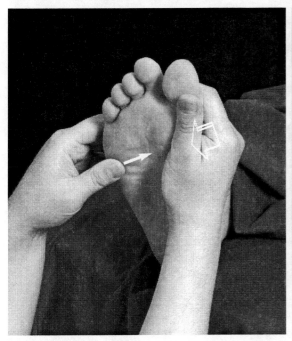

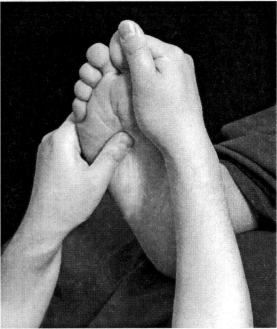

2 Place the tip of the outer (left) thumb on the outer (lateral) edge of the foot just below the ball of the foot under the smallest toe. Stroke over the outer edge of the foot by pushing the foot into the thumb with the inner hand.

3 Continue pushing the foot into the tip of the outer thumb until you reach the center of the foot.

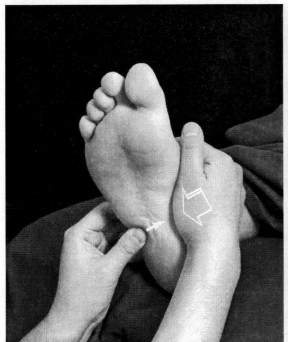

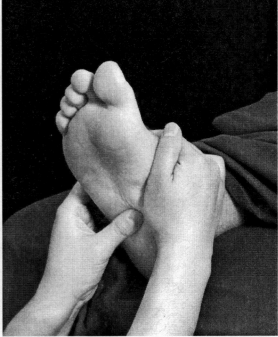

4 Move both hands down the foot one thumb-width at a time and repeat the stroke. The hands should move together so that the palm of the inner hand pushes toward the outer thumb.

5 Continue moving down and pushing the foot into your outer thumb until you reach the top edge of the heel pad. Repeat the entire sequence 2 - 3 times on each foot.

Japanese Basic Foot Massage Techniques - Example #27

Thumb Stroking Up on the Edges of the Feet

Japanese name of this technique

母指軽擦法

Bo Shi Kei Satsu Ho

The purpose of this technique

Loosen the muscles and tendons on the (lateral) edge of the foot

Where it is applied

On the (lateral) edges of the feet, excluding the toes and heels

About this technique

This technique uses deep, slow thumb stroking on the outer (lateral) edge of the foot. As with Examples #17 or #19 you stroke by pushing the foot into the thumb with the supporting hand, instead of using the thumb for the actual stroking movement. Slight lubrication is necessary, but it is a very unstable region and too much lubricant will make it difficult to stay on the edge of the foot.

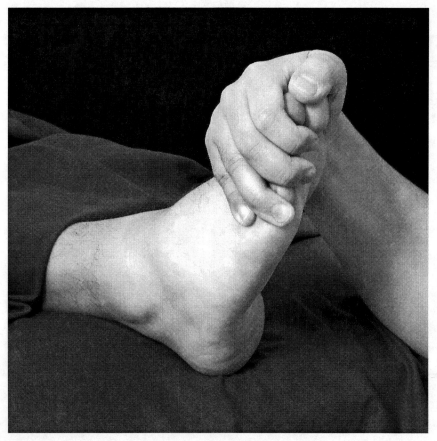

1 Grasp the top (dorsal) of the foot with your inner (right) hand. The ball of the thumb should be against the big toe and your fingers should wrap around the toes.

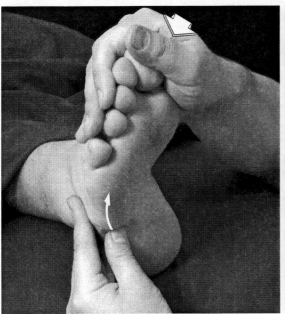

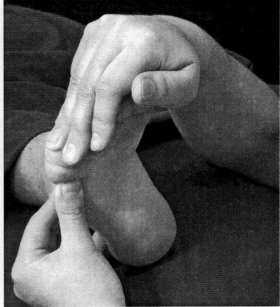

Stroking on the bottom edge of the foot:

2 Place the outer (left) thumb just above the heel pad on the outside (lateral) edge of the bottom of the foot. Push the foot down into the thumb so that it strokes up toward the fifth toe.

3 Keep pushing the foot into the outer thumb, minimizing the movement of the thumb. You may need to adjust the angle of the outer wrist so that the thumb can follow the edge of the foot, but keep the thumb as stationary as possible. Repeat 2 - 5 times.

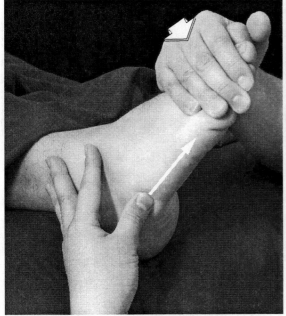

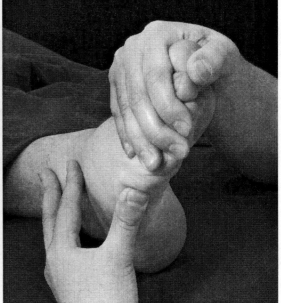

Stroking on the outer edge of the foot:

4 Keep the inner hand in the same position and place the outer thumb on the outer (lateral) edge of the foot near the heel. Push the foot into the thumb to stroke up towards the fifth toe.

5 Again, stroke by pushing the foot into the outer thumb with the inner hand, do not stroke by moving the thumb. Stop just below the fifth toe. Repeat 2 - 5 times.

Japanese Basic Foot Massage Techniques - Example #28

Stroking the Webbing of the Toes

Japanese name of this technique

二指軽擦法

Ni Shi Kei Satsu Ho

The purposes of this technique

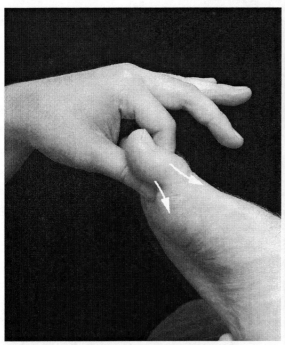

Loosen the tendons between the phalanges

Where it is applied

On the webbing between the toes and between the phalanges

About this technique

It is important to work the region between the upper foot bones (phalangeals) and over the webbing of the toes because most of the meridians of the foot run in between them. Smoothly and rhythmically stroke up and down the web with light pressure. A fair amount of lubrication will be required for smooth stroking.

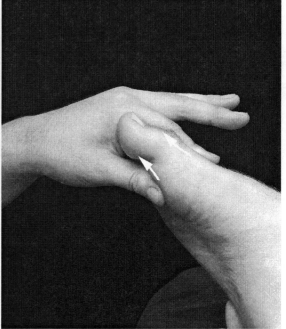

Stroking the top and bottom together:

1 Place your thumb and index finger on the webs between the first two toes. Stroke by pushing your thumb and index finger toward the ankle until the top of the toes reach the webbing of your fingers.

2 Pull with both the thumb and index finger to stroke back up until they touch at the tips. Stroke by pushing and pulling on the webbing several times. Repeat between the second and third toes and continue through each adjacent pair of toes.

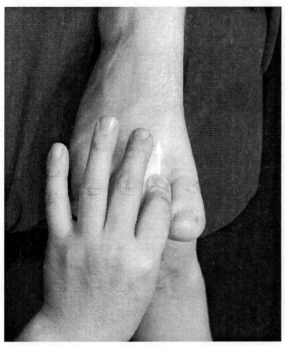

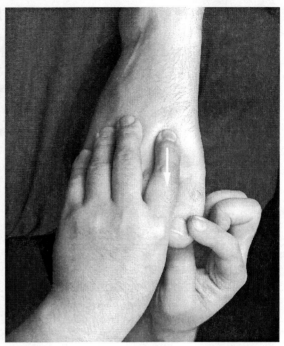

Stroking the top only:

3 Using the same finger placement as step 1 and 2, stabilize the thumb against the bottom of the web and stroke away from the toes on the top of the web with the index finger.

4 Stroke between the upper foot bones (phalangeals) as far back as you are comfortably able to stroke, then back to the thumb. Stroke up and down on the webbing several times. Repeat on the webbing between the other toes.

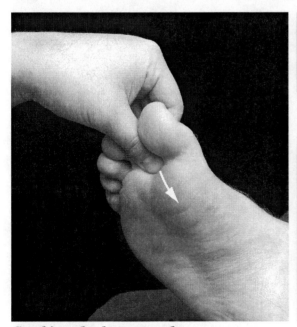

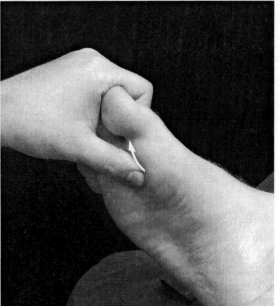

Stroking the bottom only:

5 Using the same finger placement as Steps 1 and 2, stabilize the index finger on the top of the web, stroking the bottom with the thumb.

6 This technique is the same as Steps 3 and 4, except that you are using your thumb to stroke the bottom of the web. Repeat on the webbing between the other toes.

Japanese Foot Massage Techniques - Example #29

Thumb Stroking Over the Heel

Japanese name of this technique

母指頭強擦法

Bo Shi To Kyo Satsu Ho

The purpose of this technique

Release tension on the center of the heel

Where it is applied

On the center of the heels of the feet

About this technique

This and the next example are used to work on the heel and the surrounding areas. Some people have extremely hard and/or cracked skin on the heel. Additional lubricant and slower stroking may make it easier to work under these conditions.

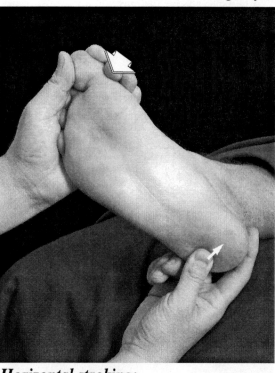
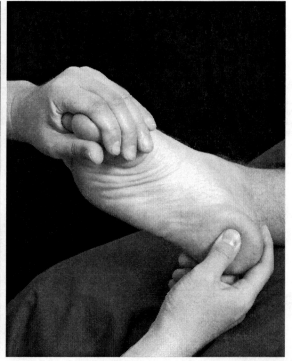

Horizontal stroking:

1 Grasp the top (dorsal) of the foot with your outer (left) hand, placing the heel of the foot between the index and middle fingers of your inner (right) hand. Place the tip of the inner thumb just to the outer (lateral) edge of the heel.

2 Keep your inner thumb straight and apply moderate to heavy pressure. Stroke across the heel horizontally with the thumb, assisting the movement by gently rotating the foot inward with the outer hand so that the big toe moves toward you. Repeat 2 - 3 times.

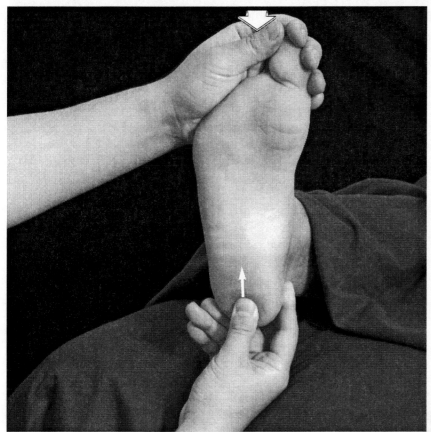

Vertical stroking:

3 Keep the outer (left) hand in the same position as steps 1 - 2. Place the tip of your inner (right) thumb on the bottom tip of the heel. Move the foot into an upright position.

4 Stroke with moderate to heavy pressure while slowly pulling the toes down toward you with the outer hand.

5 The thumb should slide over the heel as the toes are pulled toward you. Do not lift your inner wrist up to stroke the thumb upward over the heel. As you pull the toes forward, the thumb should slide slightly toward you, but be careful not to hyperextend the thumb. Stroke all the way to the upper edge of the heel pad. Repeat several times, then slightly move the thumb from left to right and continue with repeated stroking to cover the entire heel pad.

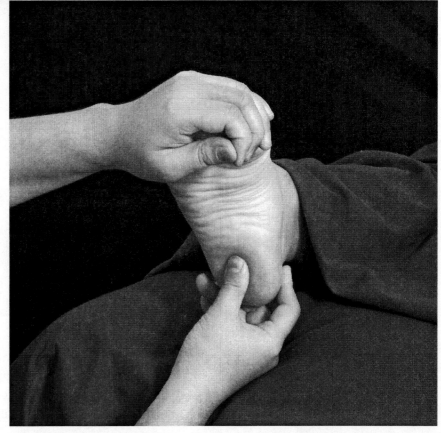

Thumb Stroking on the Edge of the Heel

Japanese name of this technique

母指頭強擦法

Bo Shi To Kyo Satsu Ho

The purpose of this technique

Reduce tension on the edges of the heel

Where it is applied

On the edges of the heels of the feet

About this technique

This technique is used to reduce tension on the edges of the heel pad. It is important that your index and middle fingers have a solid grip on the back of the heel to stabilize the hand as you stroke. It is also helpful for the outer hand to move the foot into the stroking to minimize wear on your thumb and wrist. This technique also requires a small amount of lubrication.

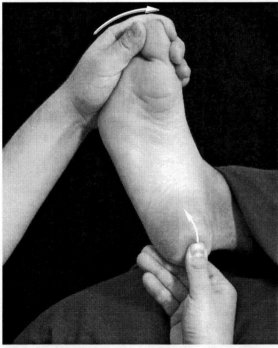
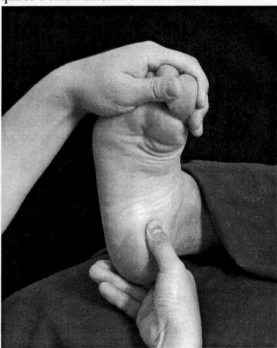

Inside (medial) edge of the heel:

1 Grasp the top (dorsal) of the foot with your outer (left) hand, placing your inner (right) index and middle fingers under the heel, and the tip of the thumb on the inside (medial) edge.

2 Apply heavy pressure with the tip of the thumb. Stroke the inside edge of the heel by gently pushing the toes inward to rotate the foot into the thumb. Repeat several times.

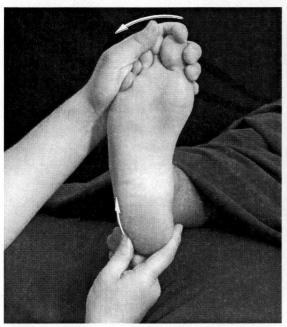

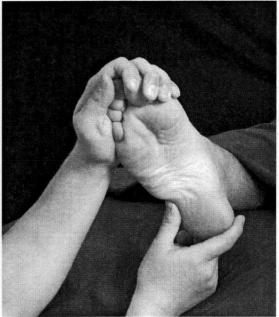

Outside (lateral) edge of the heel:

3 This is the same position as step 1, but your inner thumb is on the outside (lateral) edge of the heel. Stroke the outside edge of the heel by pulling the foot down into the thumb.

4 Continue stroking up along the outside edge of the heel with the thumb until just past the upper edge of the heel pad. Again, do not try to stroke with the thumb or lift the wrist off of the table to "assist" the stroke.

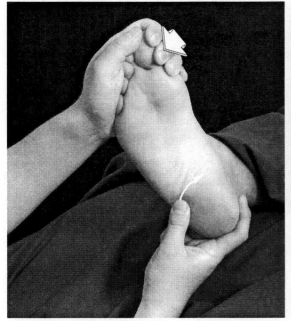

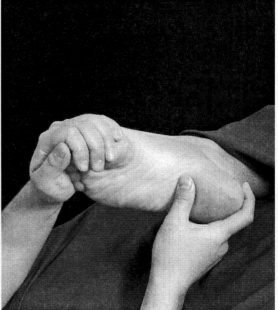

Top (anterior) edge of the heel:

5 Apply pressure by placing the thumb on the edge of the heel pad where you finished in step 4. Stroke along the top edge of the heel by rotating the foot down and toward you.

6 As you rotate the foot, the thumb will stroke toward the arch along the top edge of the heel pad. Do not bend the thumb while stroking. Repeat stroking 2 - 3 times.

Chapter Nine

JAPANESE FOOT MASSAGE TECHNIQUES

Without Lubrication

In the previous chapters I introduced thirty examples of techniques that are applied with lubrication. In this chapter, I will introduce fifteen techniques that do not require lubrication. The techniques in this chapter are from Anma (traditional Japanese massage), and not from Zoku Shin Do reflexology. The stretching techniques from Chapter 10 are also from Anma, and are easy to combine with the examples from this chapter.

You will find that these techniques are applied quite differently than the techniques from the previous chapters. If you are combining Japanese foot massage with a modality of bodywork that does not use oil such as Anma or Shiatsu, you might find these techniques easier to incorporate into your massage routine. It is both beneficial and useful to know techniques that do not use lubrication for those instances when it is not convenient. Circumstances could arise where you might not be able to work directly on a client's skin, or would prefer to avoid direct contact with the skin. Most of the techniques in this chapter can be applied over socks and still achieve stimulating results.

When you are ready to apply these techniques, it is best if you remove any lubrication with a towel before beginning. Of course, it is much easier if lubrication has not been applied at all. You can apply these techniques before the warm up techniques, but it is always best if you first warm the feet before applying deeper work. If you like, try using Examples #1 through #4 without lubrication for a quick warm up and then move to the examples in this chapter.

Most of these techniques are also easy to apply on yourself. Practicing on yourself can be a good way to feel the benefits of each technique, as well as to determine the proper amount of pressure that you should apply.

Japanese Foot Massage Techniques - Example #31

Light Kneading on the Soles of the Feet

Japanese name of this technique

母指揉揑法

Bo Shi Ju Netsu Ho

The purpose of this technique

Relax and warm the sole of the foot

Where it is applied on the feet

Over the balls and middle of the feet

About this technique

This technique uses fairly light, quick kneading to warm the foot. Unlike most kneading (Ju Netsu Ho) techniques, no rotation or kneading motion is used. It is not a pressure technique, but instead, you lightly walk down the foot with the thumbs.

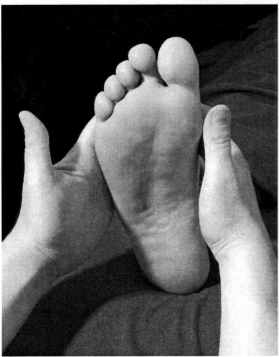

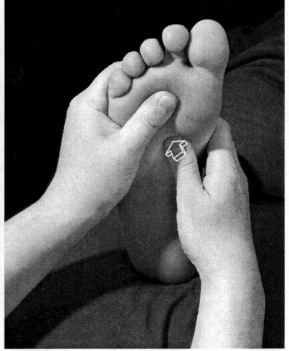

1 Place and lightly hook your fingers on the top (dorsal) of the foot, so that the index fingers are just below the base of the toes. If the foot rotates, bring it back to a straight, upright position. Bring the foot slightly toward you by relaxing your shoulders and elbows.

2 Place the inner (right) thumb on the ball of the foot under the big toe and the outer (left) thumb on the ball of the foot under the second toe. Alternate the thumbs, using light pressure to walk down the the foot. The inner thumb should follow the first foot bone (metatarsal), and the outer thumb the second.

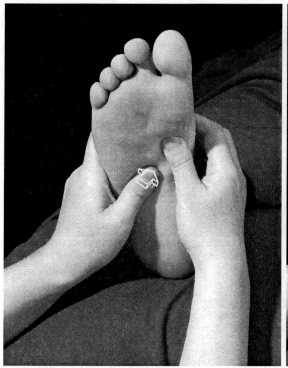

3 As you walk down the sole of the foot by alternating thumbs, each thumb should move to just below the other one.

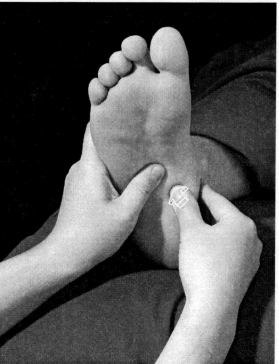

4 Continue walking down the foot, following the edge of the arch, until you reach the top of the heel pad.

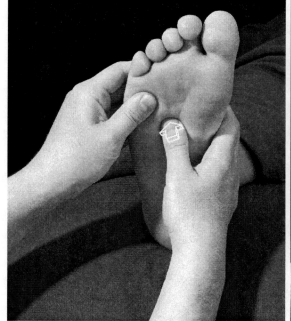

5 Move the tips of your thumbs to the ball of the foot at either the fourth and fifth or third and fifth foot bones. Again walk down the foot with the tips of the thumbs, this time along the outside edge of the bottom of the foot.

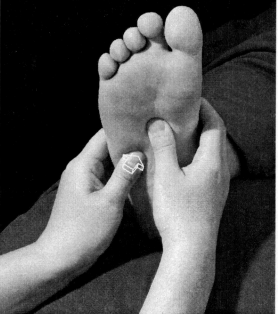

6 Continue walking down the foot until you reach the edge of the heel pad. The entire sequence should be repeated 2 - 5 times until the bottom of the foot is properly warmed. Repeat on the other foot.

Japanese Foot Massage Techniques - Example #32

Rotation on the Arches with the Heel of the Hand

Japanese names of these techniques

母指球揉捏法

Bo Shi Kyu Ju Netsu Ho
Ko Shi Kyu Ju Netsu Ho

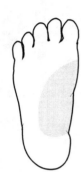

The purpose of these techniques

Reduce muscle tension and restore the conture of the arch

Where they are applied

On the arches of the feet

About these techniques

This technique looks similar to Example #24, but it uses small rotations by gripping the skin without lubricant, instead of sliding over the skin with lubricant. Two different ways to apply this technique are shown. To minimize stress to the wrist, you may choose to use the base of the thumb (thenar), base of the side of the hand (hypothenar), or both sides to work on the arch, depending on the angle and size of the client's foot and the size of your hands. Rotation must come from shoulder movement and not from the wrist.

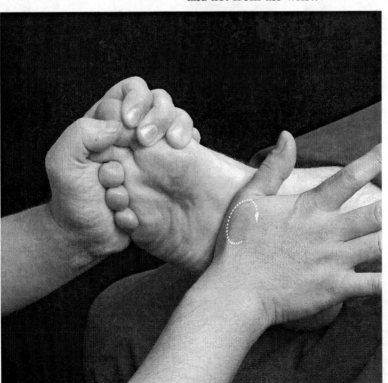

Base of the thumb:

1 Grasp the top of the foot by wrapping the fingers of your outer (left) hand around the big toe to stabilize the foot. Place the base of the thumb (thenar side) of your inner (right) hand in the arch of the foot.

2 Apply small rotations with fairly heavy pressure, minimizing movement over the surface of the skin. Remember to rotate from the shoulder, not from the wrist. Cover the entire arch on each foot.

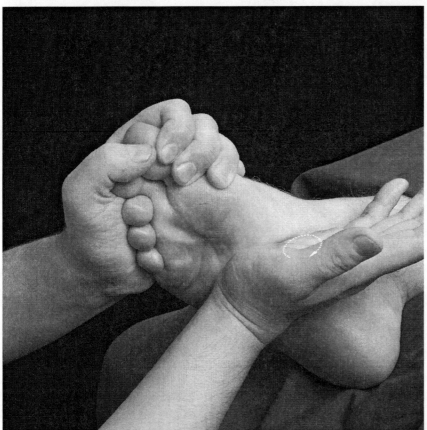

Base of the side of the hand:

3 This uses the same concept as the previous variation, but it is applied with the other side of the hand. Again, stabilize the foot with your outer hand. Place the base of the side of the inner hand (hypothenar) on the arch of the foot. To avoid sliding the hand over the skin, apply a fair amount of pressure and use small rotations.

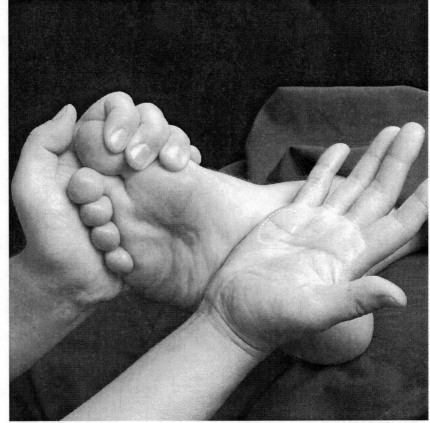

4 Cover the entire arch region from just above the heel pad to just below the ball of the foot under the big toe. Adjust the angle of the hand to the conture of the arch for the best fit. Repeat on the other foot using either or both variations.

Japanese Foot Massage Techniques - Example #33

Roll Over the Arches with the Tip of the Thumb

Japanese name of this technique

母指頭揉捏法

Bo Shi To Ju Netsu Ho

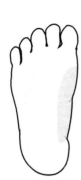

The purpose of this technique

Reduce the muscle tension on the arch of the foot

Where it is applied on the feet

Inside (medial) edge of the longitudinal arches

About this technique

This technique is an effective way to loosen tight muscles on the arches. Use a fair amount of pressure to be both effective and therapeutic. Although the therapeutic level will cause your client to experience slight discomfort, avoid using excessive pressure that could cause too much discomfort. The majority of movement is done by using the outer hand (the hand on the toes) to move the foot left and right, minimizing stress to the thumb.

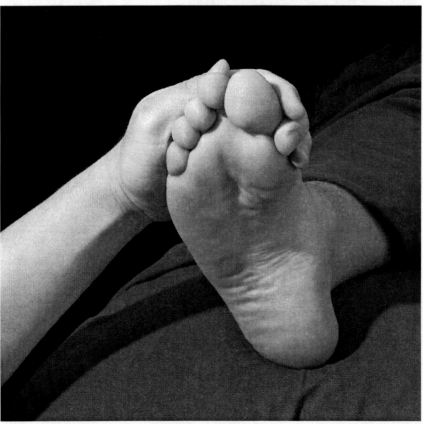

1 Cup the top (dorsal) of the foot with your outer (left) hand over the toes. Make sure that the tips of the fingers and ball of the thumb have a firm grip on either side of the top of the foot.

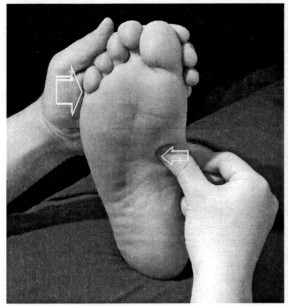

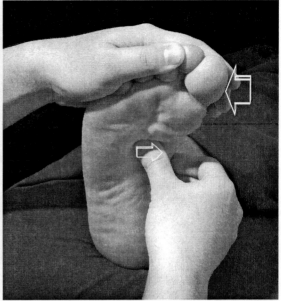

2 Place the fingers of the inner (right) hand near the inner ankle for support, applying pressure with the tip of the thumb to the arch, just below the ball of the foot under the big toe. With the outer hand, push the foot inward, stopping after the inner thumb rolls across the first metatarsal.

3 Maintain firm thumb pressure and roll back over the arch by pulling the foot outward with the outer hand. Slowly knead the muscle by rolling back and forth over the arch, sliding with the skin over the bone. Do not slide the thumb over the surface of the skin.

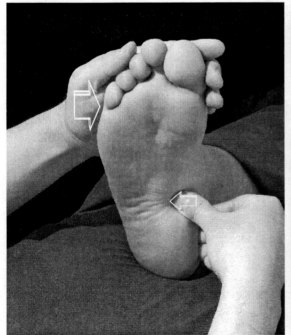

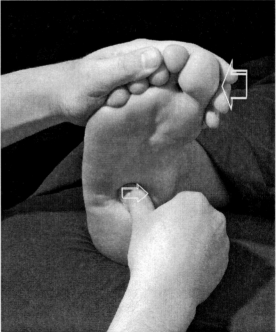

4 Roll over the arch 3 - 5 times, repeating as you move toward the heel one thumb-width at a time.

5 Work down the arch (moving past the 1st metatarsal to the 1st cuneiform and navicular bones) stopping just above the heel pad. Repeat on the other foot.

Japanese Foot Massage Techniques - Example #34

Kneading the Middles of the Feet

Japanese name of this technique

母指揉捏法

Bo Shi Ju Netsu Ho

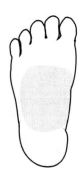

The purpose of this technique

Reduce the muscle tension of the middle of the foot

Where it is applied on the feet

On the middle of the feet

About this technique

This technique kneads the muscle by applying pressure with the thumbs, alternating one after the other. The concept of this technique is commonly used in Ko Ho Anma (traditional Japanese massage) such as when kneading the erector muscles. Wipe away any lubrication, and use heavy enough pressure so that you will be able to work into the foot with your thumbs without slippage. This technique should be applied by moving from your upper body, not just with the thumbs.

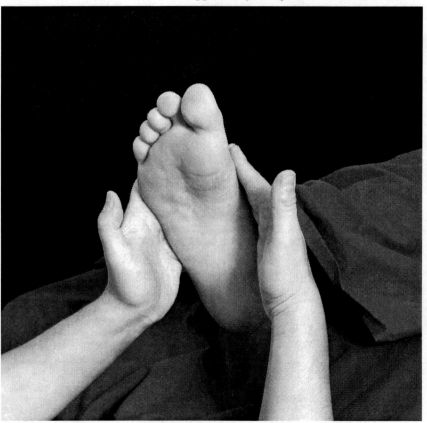

1 Place the fingertips of the inner (right) hand over the first foot bone (metatarsal) on the top (dorsal) of the foot and the fingertips of the outer (left) hand over the fifth foot bone.

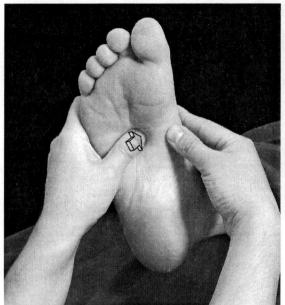

2 Place the tips of both thumbs just below the ball of the foot under the big toe, on either side of the arch. With the outer (left) thumb, apply medium to deep pressure into the foot and slightly toward the inner (medial) edge so that the muscle is pushed toward the inner (right) thumb.

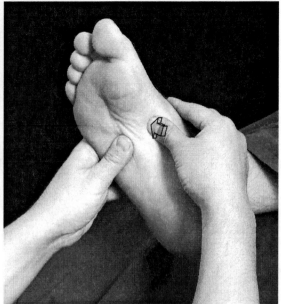

3 Apply pressure with the inner thumb, pushing the muscle toward the outer thumb. Release pressure of the outer thumb as soon as the muscle pushes against it. Keep kneading slowly down the arch, alternating the thumbs until you reach the upper edge of the heel pad.

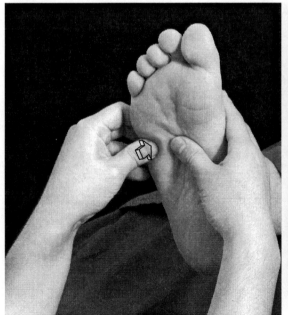

4 Move the thumbs to the outside (lateral) edge of the foot, placing both thumbs just below either side of the ball of the foot under the smallest toe and repeat the kneading process of Step 2 - 3.

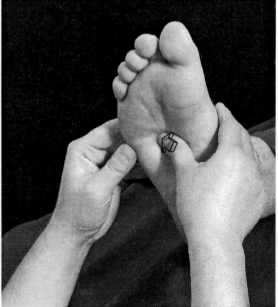

5 Continue kneading the outside edge of the foot while slowly moving downward until you reach the upper edge of the heel pad. Repeat on the other foot.

Japanese Foot Massage Techniques - Example #35

Kneading the Heels with the Thumbs

Japanese name of this technique

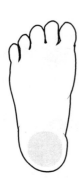

母指揉捏法

Bo Shi Ju Netsu Ho

The purpose of this technique

Loosen the muscles and ligaments of the heel

Where it is applied on the feet

On the heels

About this technique

This uses the same concept as the previous technique, except that
it is applied on the heel. The surface of the heel can be much
harder than other surfaces of the foot. Make sure that the foot is
firmly stabilized with the fingers of both hands. Any lubrication
must be removed, or this technique will be difficult to apply.
The prone position, especially when working from the end of the
table, is also a very effective way to work on the heel of the foot.

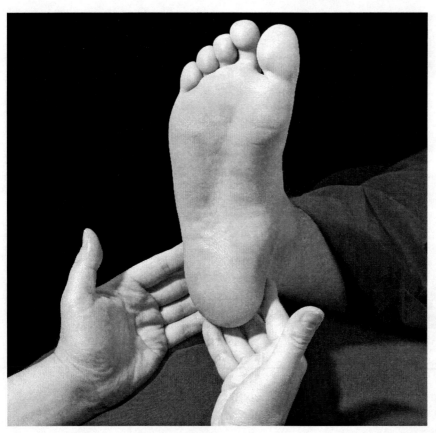

1 Support the heel
with the tips of the
fingers of both hands.
Place the middle fin-
gers behind either side
of the ankle. Bring
the foot into as
upright a position as
possible.

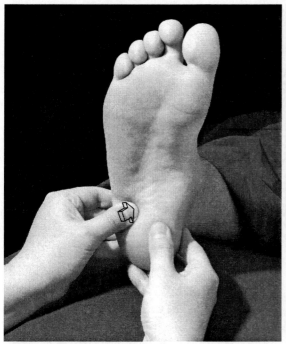

2 Place the thumbs at a 45° angle to the top edge of the heel pad, about one thumb-width apart. Apply strong inward, and slightly upward pressure with the outer (left) thumb.

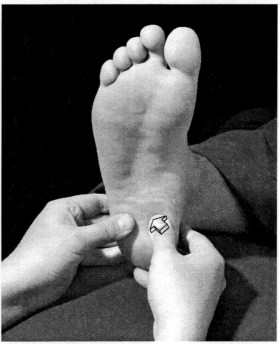

3 Apply pressure toward the outer thumb with the inner (right) thumb. Release pressure of the outer thumb as soon as the muscle pushes against it. Knead by alternating the thumbs.

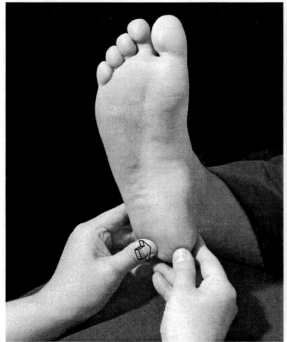

4 After repeating several times, move the thumbs down one thumb-width at a time and continue kneading. Repeat several times.

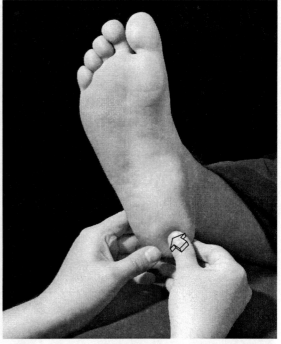

5 Continue moving down with alternating thumbs until you reach the bottom edge of the heel pad. Repeat on the other heel.

Japanese Foot Massage Techniques - Example #36

Thumb Rotation on the Middles of the Feet

Japanese name of this technique

母指揉揑法

Bo Shi Kei Satsu Ho

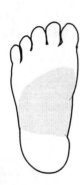

The purpose of this technique

Loosen the muscles on the middle of the foot

Where it is applied

Middles of the feet in between the heel and the ball

About this technique

This technique is most often used to work the middle of the foot. It can also be used to work the balls of the foot between the metatarsals and the phalanges. Again, keep your thumb almost stationary, and rotate by using the outer hand to move the foot into the thumb to minimize stress to your thumb. **Do not rotate the inner thumb.** The thumb should remain in contact with the same place during the rotation, and should not slide over the surface of the skin.

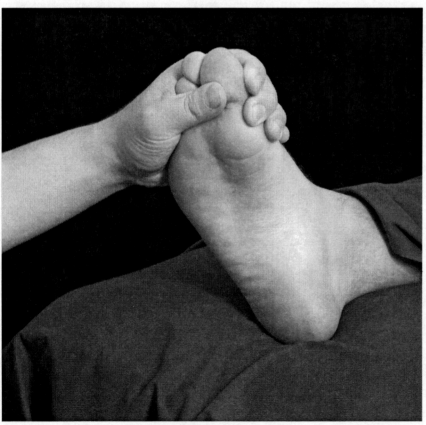

1 Grasp the top of the foot over the toes with your outer (left) hand and rotate the foot slightly for better access to the middle of the foot.

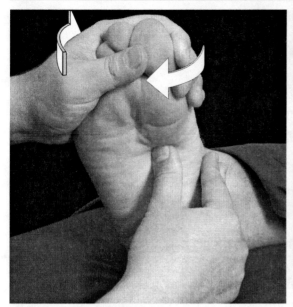

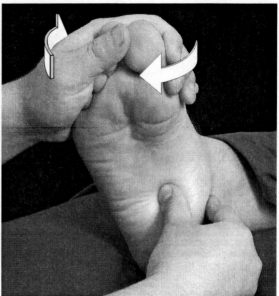

2 Place the tip of the inner (right) thumb just below the ball of the foot under the big toe and pull the foot gently into the thumb.
Slightly rotate the foot with the outer hand into the thumb, circling once every few seconds.
Do not rotate the thumb, movement is made by the outer hand.

3 Move the inner thumb about one thumb-width toward the heel between the first and second foot bones (metatarsals). Apply pressure and rotate as you did in step 2. Continue moving down the foot one thumb width at a time stopping at the top edge of the heel pad.

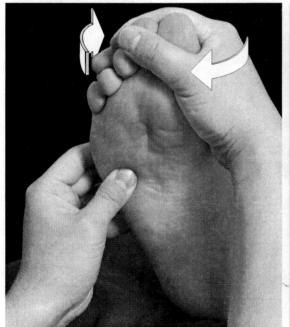

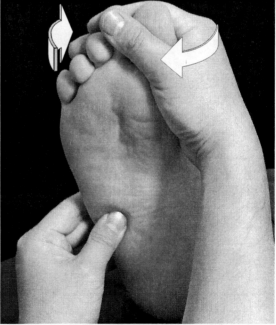

4 Move between the next set of foot bones and repeat the rotations as you did in steps 2 - 3. Cover the area from just below the ball of the foot under each toe, to the top edge of the heel pad.

5 Repeat between each set of foot bones. For the 3rd - 5th foot bones, it may be easier to switch hands, using the inner hand for rotation and the outer hand for pressure on each foot.

Japanese Foot Massage Techniques - Example #37

Two Thumb Kneading On the Arches

Japanese name of this technique

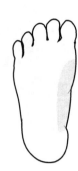

母指揉捏法

Bo Shi Ju Netsu Ho

The purpose of this technique

Reduce muscle tension and increase flexibility along the arch

Where it is applied on the feet

On the inner (medial) edge of the arches of the feet (over the first metatarsal, the first cuneiform, and navicular bones)

About this technique

This thumb pressure technique is similar to Example #34, although it is applied with both thumbs on the same side of muscle instead of on either side of it. The outer hand (the hand over the toes) can gently stretch the big toe while applying this technique to increase effectiveness. Make sure that you adjust the amount of pressure according to the sensitivity of your client. **Do not bend the thumb, the thumb should be kept straight while applying pressure.**

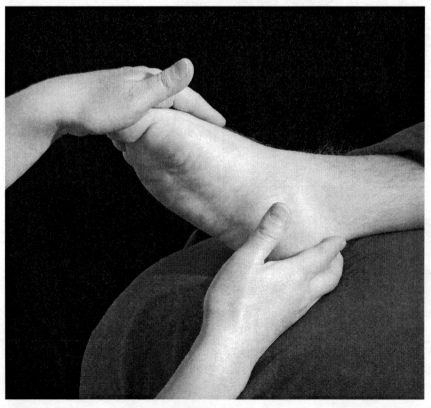

1 Place the outer (left) hand gently on the top (dorsal) of the foot over the toes so that that the big toe is touching the ball of the thumb. Lightly hook the fingers of the inner (right) hand beneath the heel for stability.

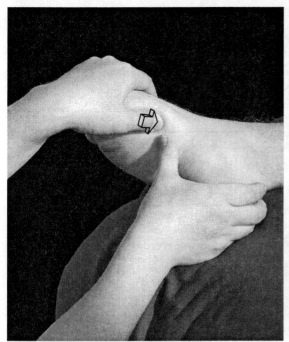

2 Place your thumbs side by side on the inside (medial) edge of the first foot bone (metatarsal) just below the ball of the foot under the big toe. Apply strong pressure with the tip of the outer thumb.

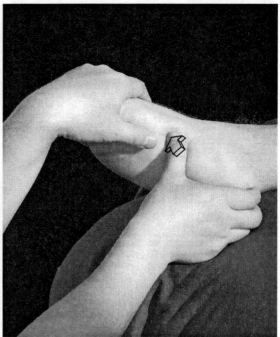

3 Apply strong pressure with the tip of the inner thumb as the outer one releases pressure. Alternate thumb pressure, slightly overlapping the region of application.

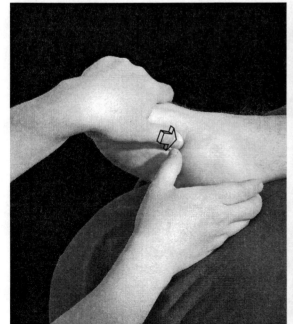

4 Alternate thumbs to create a kneading movement. With each alternation, the thumbs should move slightly toward the heel along with the inside (medial) edge of the first foot bones.

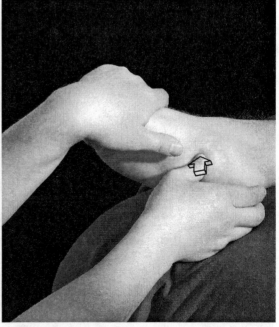

5 Continue kneading until you reach the edge of the heel pad. The pressure should come from using upper body movement, not just from the hands. Repeat 2 - 3 times on each foot.

Fan Kneading the Balls of the Feet

Japanese name of this technique

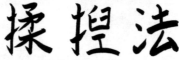

Ju NetsuHo

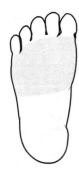

The purpose of this technique

Increase flexibility and loosen tight muscles and ligaments

Where it is applied on the feet

On the balls of the feet

About this technique

This is a very old Anma (Ko Ho Anma) technique and is actually very simple even though it may look complicated. It is excellent for loosening tight muscles and ligaments around the balls of the feet. The application of this technique should come from movement of your upper body, not just from moving your hands and wrists. **Do not bend the thumb during this technique.** Again, make sure that you adjust to the sensitivity of each client.

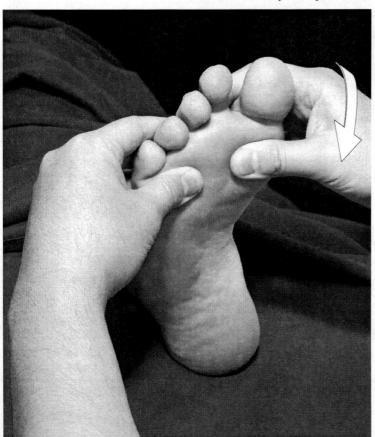

1 Place the fingers of your inner (right) hand over the second foot bone (metatarsal) on the top (dorsal) of the foot, so that the index finger is at the base of the second toe. Place the fingers of outer (left) hand over the fourth foot bone, so that the index finger is at the base of the fourth toe. Place the inner thumb on the center of the ball of the foot under the big toe, and the outer thumb on the center of the ball of the foot under the smallest toe.

2 Begin pulling downward and toward you with your inner hand, using the thumb as leverage. This stretches the big toe and the inner (medial) side of the top of the foot.

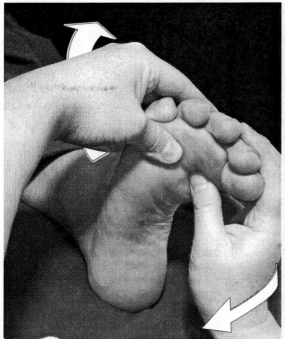

3 Continue to pull the inner side toward you as far as is comfortable for the client, while using the thumb of the outer hand to push the outer (lateral) side of the foot away from you.

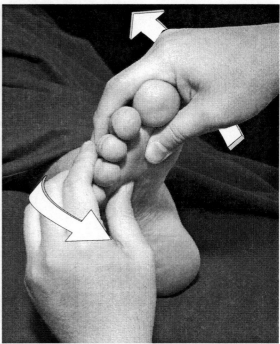

4 Rotate the inner side of the top of the foot by using the inner thumb to push away from you, while using the outer hand to start pulling the outer side of the foot toward you.

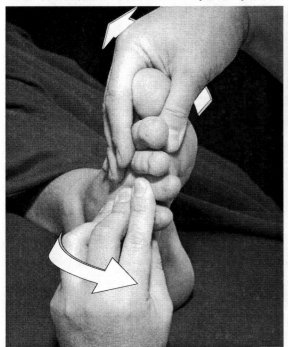

5 Continue to pull the outer side of the top of the foot toward you, while pushing the inner side of the foot away from you as far as is comfortable for the client.

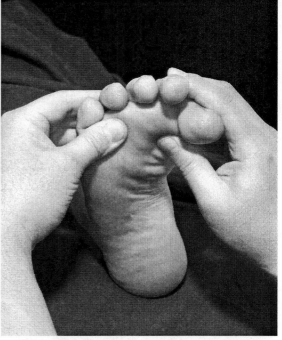

6 Continue the fanning movement as you return to the beginning position and bring the inner hand back toward you while pushing away from you with the outer hand. Repeat for about 30 seconds on each foot.

Japanese Foot Massage Techniques - Example #39

Vibration on the Feet

Japanese names of these techniques

振せん法

Bo Shi To Shin Sen Ho (step 1-2)
Shu Ken Shin Sen Ho (step 3-5)

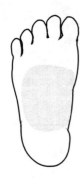

The purpose of these techniques

Help loosen tight areas on the foot, especially deep layers

Where they are applied on the feet

Middle of the feet and surrounding regions

About these techniques

These vibration techniques can be combined at any time with any of the other techniques. Typically, I use it briefly as a transition technique between two others or in the middle of one to aid in loosening. For example, you could combine thumb stroking and rotation with vibration, or knuckle stroking with vibration. You can use any part of the hand to do vibration, depending on which part of your hand best fits in the curvature of the foot. Always apply direct pressure or press firmly against the foot first, and then vibrate. You can use both inner or outer vibration (see p. 70) for most of the techniques shown here, but inner vibration will produce the best results.

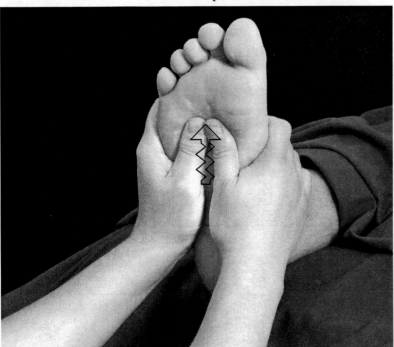

Vibration with Thumbs:

1 Grasp the foot firmly in both hands so that your thumbs are on the soles of the foot and the fingers are on the top (dorsal) side of the foot.

2 Apply pressure with the thumbs to the center of the foot, or wherever else you desire, using your fingers for leverage. Vibration is created by vibrating your shoulders and arms with the hands. You can use either one or both thumbs to apply the vibration.

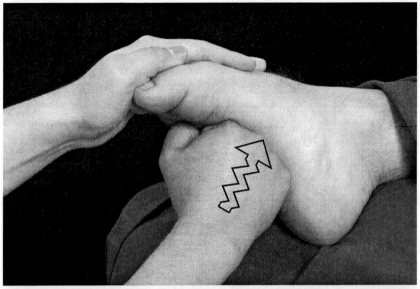

Vibration with the flat part of fist:

3 Make a fist with your inner (right) hand and place the flat part into the arch. Wrap the outer (left) hand over the toes and top of the foot. Firmly stabilize the fist and pull the outer hand downward into the fist, then vibrate the fist from your shoulder and arm.

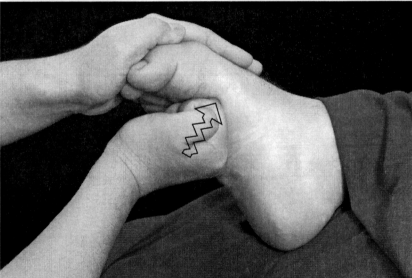

Vibration with the tips of the knuckles:

4 This is similar to the previous variation, but you need to rotate your wrist 90° and use the tips of the fist instead of the flat part. Firmly stabilize the fist and pull the outer hand downward into the knuckles, then vibrate the fist from your shoulder and arm.

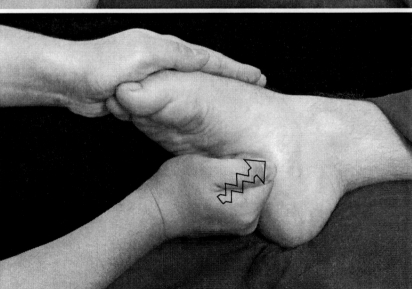

5 Move slightly down toward the heel, continuing the vibration until just above the heel pad. As you get closer to the heel, you will need to more firmly stabilize the wrist, because it becomes difficult to sustain a firm application into the arch.

Japanese Foot Massage Techniques - Example #40

Forearm and Elbow Vibration in the Arches

Japanese names of these techniques

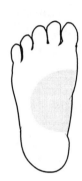

肘頭振せん法

Zen Wan Shin Sen Ho
Chu To Shin Sen Ho

The purpose of these techniques

Reduce tension on the arch, especially deep layers

Where they are applied on the feet

In the arches of the feet

About these techniques

Here I will introduce two applications of this technique. You can choose between them depending on what seems to be the most appropriate. Not everybody is able to apply smooth vibration. Beginners may find it easier to vibrate by using the forearm or the tip of the elbow. You can either use inner vibration or outer vibration (see p. 70), whichever feels most comfortable.

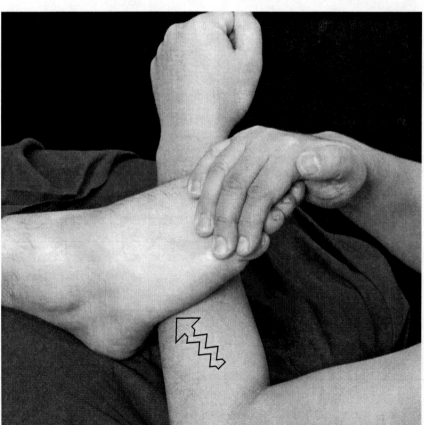

Forearm (Zen Wan Shin Sen Ho):

1 Rest the elbow of your outer (left) arm against the table. Place the inner (right) hand on top (dorsal) of the foot and press the foot against your arm, so that the toes wrap over your forearm. The arm must be firmly supported.

2 Push the foot down into the forearm with the inner hand. Tense the forearm and fist of the outer hand and vibrate the arm for about 3 - 7 seconds. Repeat as desired.

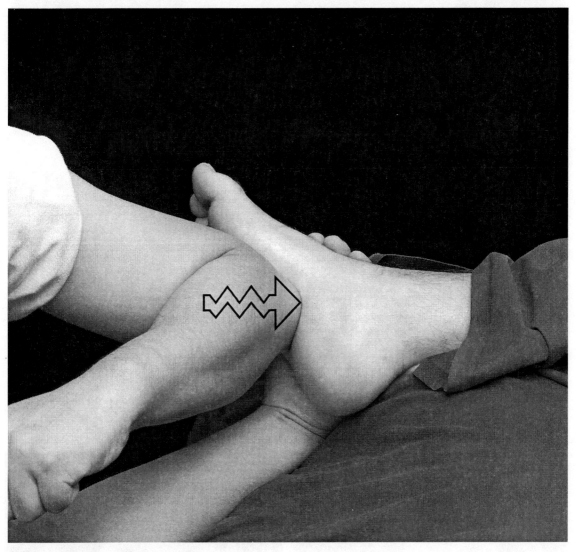

Elbow (Chu To Shin Sen Ho):

This vibration is applied with stronger stimulation than the previous application. Lubrication should be removed from the foot to avoid slippage. If it is difficult to remove lubricant, you can wrap a sheet around the foot, then apply this technique.

3 Grasp the foot with your inner (right) hand so that the palm is over the ankle, the fingers are wrapped firmly over the top (dorsal) of the foot, and the thumb is over the achilles tendon. If necessary, slightly rotate the foot outward for better access to the arch.

4 Place the tip of the elbow of your outer (left) arm on the region of the arch where you wish to apply vibration, so that the foot is firmly supported between the elbow and the inner hand. Tense the elbow and fist, vibrating the arm from the shoulder while pushing the elbow toward the inner hand. Vibration should last between 3 - 7 seconds. Move up or down the arch as you desire.

Japanese Foot Massage Techniques - Example #41

Percussion on the Feet

Japanese names of these techniques

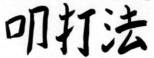

Ko Da Ho

The purpose of these techniques

Increase circulation and release muscle tension in the foot

Where they are applied

On the balls and in the middle of the feet

About these techniques

Like vibration, percussion can be used at any time during the course of a foot massage, either with or without lubrication. There are many different variations of percussion that can be used on the feet. Here I will demonstrate the three most common percussion techniques for the feet. Percussion techniques can be used to provide good transitions between other techniques. With all percussion techniques, make sure the wrist remains very loose.

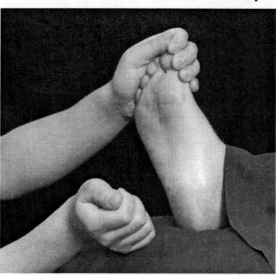

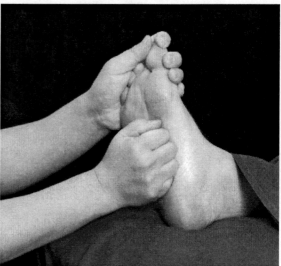

Lightly closed fist (*Shu Ken Ko Da Ho*):

1 Grasp the top (dorsal) of the foot with your outer (left) hand and rotate the foot slightly to expose the arch for percussion. Make a loose fist with the inner (right) hand and use the backs of the fingers over the knuckles to strike the foot for the percussion.

2 Strike lightly and rapidly. This is usually used on the middle of the foot, but it can be applied over most regions of the foot. Make sure to keep your hand and wrist loose to soften the impact.

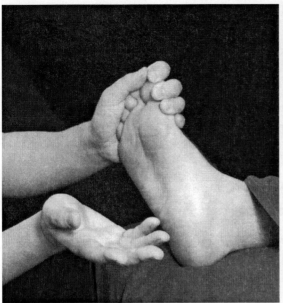
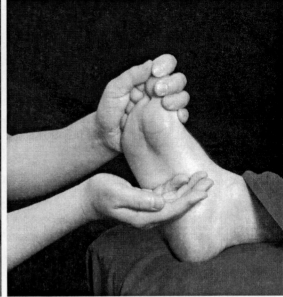

Side of the hand *(Setsu Da Ho)*:

3 Maintain the same outer hand position as steps 1 - 2. Open the inner hand so that it is loose and relaxed, applying percussion by using the inner (medial) edges of the middle, ring, and pinky fingers to contact the foot.

4 Strike quickly and lightly while slowly moving up and down the arch to cover the entire region. Because of its smaller contact surface, this technique works especially well for smaller feet.

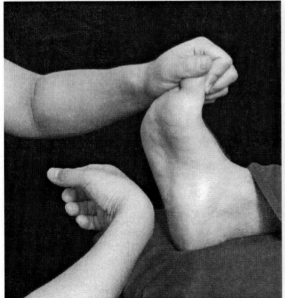
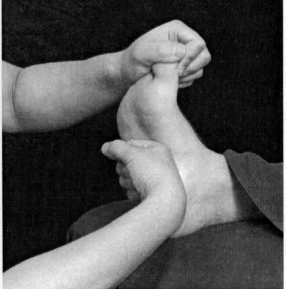

Back of the hand *(Shu Hai Ko Da Ho)*:

5 Use the same outer hand position as in steps 1 - 4, except that here you will lightly push the toes back to expose and extend the arch of the foot. Make a loose fist with the inner hand and use the back of the hand to strike the foot.

6 Strike smoothly and rhythmically as you slowly move up and down to cover the entire arch. This variation provides much deeper stimulation because it hits the surface of the foot harder. Apply for about ten seconds or as desired for each foot.

Japanese Foot Massage Techniques - Example #42

Percussion on the Edges of the Feet

Japanese name of this technique

母指叩打法

Bo Shi Ko Da Ho

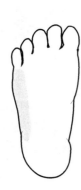

The purpose of this technique

Loosen the muscles on the outside (lateral) edge of the foot

Where it is applied on the feet

Outside (lateral) edges of the feet

About this technique

This technique is different from the rest of the percussion techniques. It is applied by almost stroking the edge of the foot and letting the foot "fall" to be caught by the web between the thumb and index finger. It may take a little practice for you to apply smoothly and rhythmically. The elbow and shoulder should remain relaxed during application of the percussion. Traction is very important, so lubrication should be removed to maintain optimum effectiveness for this techinique.

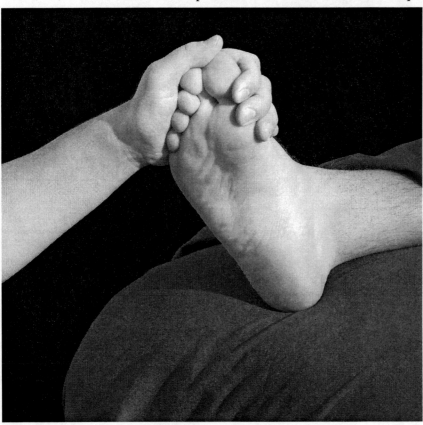

1 Grasp the top (dorsal) of the foot with your outer (left) hand. The ball of the thumb should wrap around the top of the toes.

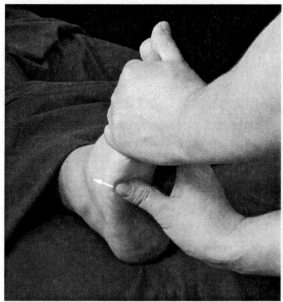

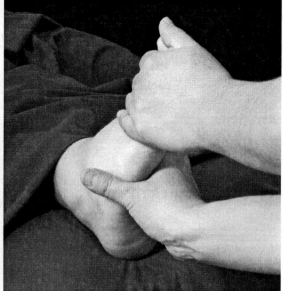

2 Place your inner (right) thumb on the foot just under the ball of the foot below the smallest toe. You should feel the hump of muscle and tendon which runs along the outside (lateral) edge of the foot. Apply strong pressure with the inner thumb. **Do not bend the thumb during this technique**, the thumb should be kept straight.

3 Slightly rotate the foot into the thumb with the outer hand. The thumb will automatically slide off the edge of the foot and fall into the inner hand to be caught by the web between the thumb and index finger. You should feel the snap, as the webbing catches the outside edge of the foot for the percussion. This is a vigorous application.

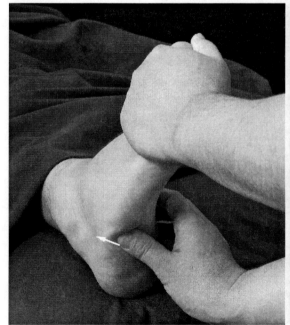

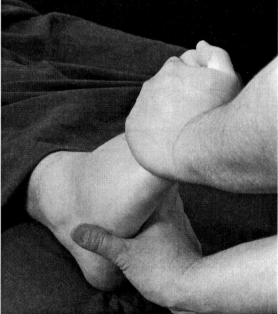

4 Keep moving down one thumb-width at a time toward the heel with each percussion.

5 Continue until you reach the top of the heel pad. You can repeat the entire procedure several times as desired. Repeat on the other foot.

Japanese Foot Massage Techniques - Example #43

Two Finger Rotation on the Tops of the Feet

Japanese name of this technique

二指揉捏法

Ni Shi Ju Netsu Ho

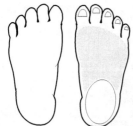

The purpose of this technique

Reduce muscle tension and increase ki flow on top of the foot

Where it is applied on the feet

Top side (dorsal) of the feet

About this technique

This example is one of the few techniques in this book that shows how to work on the top (dorsal) of the foot. This technique applies rotation to the top of the foot with the middle and ring fingers. Apply pressure gradually because some regions can tolerate a lot of pressure, while others can be very sensitive. The area of application is fairly large, so take your time and cover the entire area. You can either alternate hands, or you can alternate to use the index and middle fingers to avoid tiring either the hands or fingers.

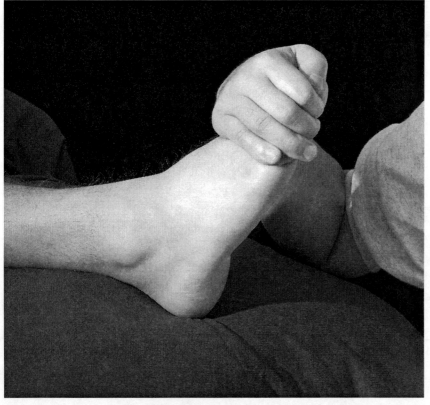

1 Grasp the top (dorsal) of the foot around the toes with your inner (right) hand for support. Pull the foot slightly downward and toward you for better access to the top of the foot and for finger placement.

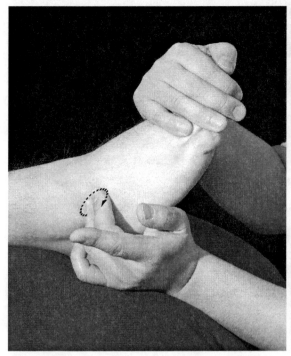

2 Hook the middle and ring finger of the outer (left) hand, slightly overlapping, just in front of the ankle on the top of the foot. Use the weight of your arm to pull toward you. **Rotate by using the entire hand, not just the fingers.**

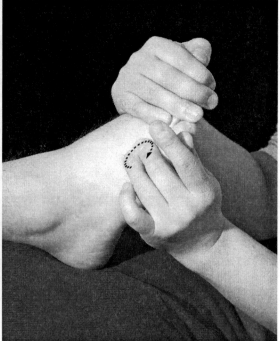

3 As you rotate, slowly slide the fingers toward the toes. Stay between the foot bones (metatarsals) and work all the way to the base of the toes. Repeat between the next set of foot bones.

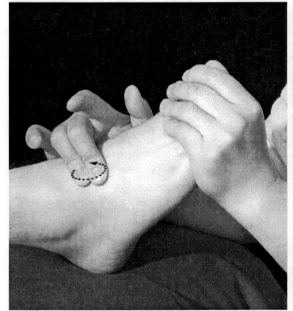

4 For the medial half of the foot, it is easier to switch your hand placements and apply rotations with the index and ring fingers of the inner hand. Rotate as in steps 2 and 3.

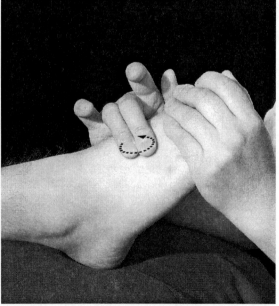

5 After you reach the base of the toes, move to the the hollow between the first and second foot bones and continue rotations. Once you have covered entire top of the foot, repeat on the other foot

Japanese Foot Massage Techniques - Example #44

Rotation and Kneading the Toes

Japanese name of these techniques

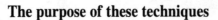

Ni Shi Ju Netsu Ho
Bo Shi Ju Netsu Ho

The purpose of these techniques

Reduce muscle tension on the toes

Where they are applied on the feet

On the toes, both top and bottom (dorsal and plantar) sides

About these techniques

I introduced techniques for working on toes in Example #7, but this will work the muscles at a much deeper level. The bottom (plantar) side of the toe is massaged using the same concept as Example #34. This technique can be applied with lubricant, but is easier and more effective without it.

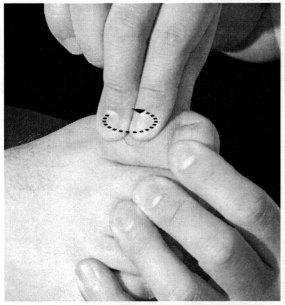
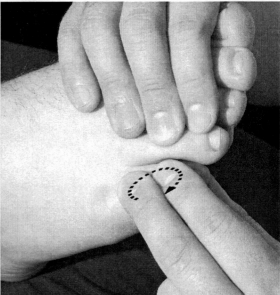

Two finger rotation on the top of the toes:

1 Place the slightly overlapped index and middle fingers of the inner (right) hand together to grasp the big toe with the thumb. Lightly grasp the other toes with the outer (left) hand for support. Apply pressure with the index and middle fingers and rotate 5 - 10 times.

2 Move to the second toe and repeat step 1, working each toe in succession. For the third through the fifth toes, it may be easier to work by switching hands. Apply just enough pressure so that you do not slip over the surface of the skin, but do not squeeze too hard.

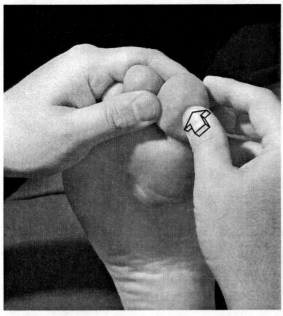 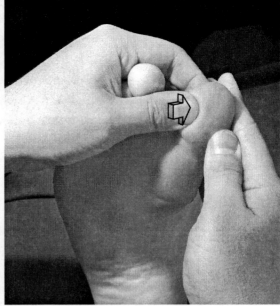

Two thumb kneading on the bottom of the toes:

3 Grasp the big toe between the index fingers and thumbs of both hands. Your thumbs should be slightly apart on the ball of the toe. Firmly support the toe with the index fingers as you press into the toe with the inner thumb.

4 Apply pressure with the outer thumb toward the index finger of the inner hand. Release the pressure with the inner thumb as soon as the big toe pushes against it. Knead the big toe by alternating thumbs.

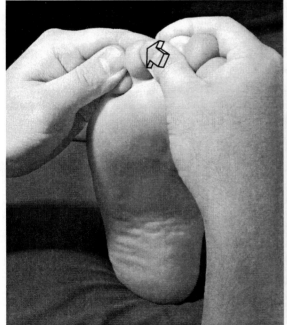 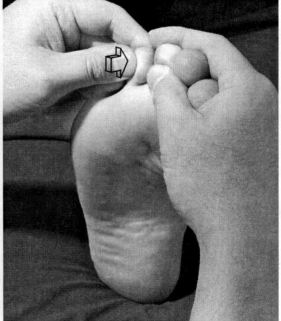

5 Move to the second toe and repeat steps 3 - 4. Always keep the index and middle fingers of both hands behind the toe for support during pressure, and also to protect against hyperextending the toe backward.

6 Continue moving down the toes, one at a time, repeating steps 3 - 4 until you reach the smallest toe. Use smaller thumb movements for the smaller toes to help stay on the toes. Repeat on the other foot.

Japanese Foot Massage Techniques - Example #45

Apply Pressure to Tsubo on the Soles of the Feet

Japanese name of this technique

母指壓迫法

Bo Shi Ap Paku Ho

The purpose of this technique

Enhance and maintain good health by stimulating tsubo

Where it is applied on the feet

Soles of the feet, at points listed individually in example

About this technique

This last example stimulates tsubos (acupoints) which are important points on the foot to enhance and maintain good overall health. Two of the tsubo are Ki Ketsu (extraordinary points, see pp. 31 - 32) and do not belong to any of the Keiraku (Meridian systems). It is best to apply pressure while the client is exhaling. Repeat three times on each point for each foot. Adjust the amount of pressure according to the client's sensitivity.

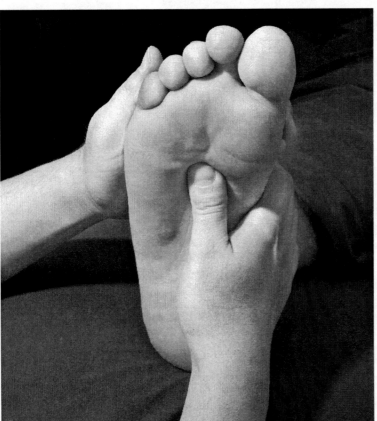

Yu Sen (Kidney #1):

Yu Sen literally means "gushing spring" or "bubbling fountain." It is the first tsubo on the Kidney meridian and is very important for maintaining good health.

1 Grasp the top (dorsal) of the foot with your outer (left) hand for support. Place the tip of the inner (right) thumb on Yu Sen. It is usually sensitive, so apply pressure gradually.

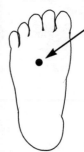

Yu Sen
This tsubo is found in the middle of the foot, in between the 2nd and 3rd foot bones (metatarsals) (see p. 42).

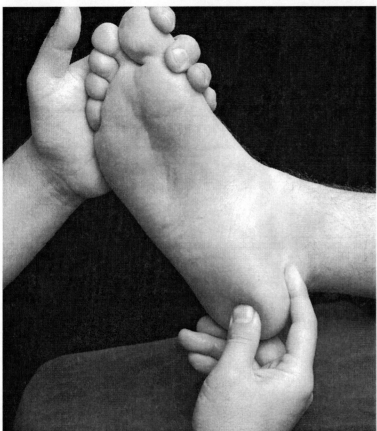

Shitsu Min (*Extraordinary point*):

Shitsu Min or "loosing sleep" is used to promote good sleep and help insomniacs.

2 Grasp and stabilize the top of foot with your outer hand. Place the index and middle fingers of the inner hand around the heel for support, placing the tip of the thumb at Shitsu Min (see below). Apply pressure with the thumb while the client slowly exhales.

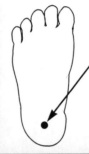

Shitsu Min
This point is found directly in the center of the heel pad on the sole of the foot.

Zoku Shin (*Extraordinary point*):

Zoku Shin literally means "heart of feet" or "center of feet"

3 Grasp and support the top of the foot with the fingers of both hands. Place the tips of the thumbs, one on top of the other at Zoku Shin. Apply pressure with both thumbs. Again, it is best to apply while the client slowly exhales.

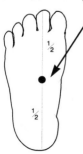

Zoku Shin
This point is found exactly at the midpoint of the sole of the foot between the tip of the second toe and bottom of the heel.

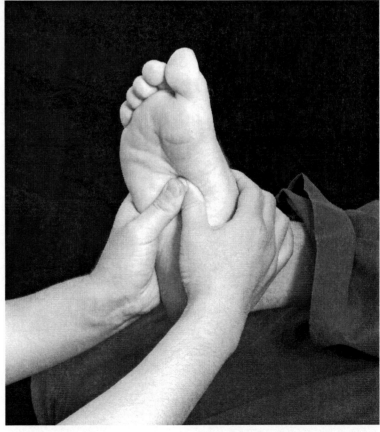

Chapter Ten

FOOT STRETCHING TECHNIQUES

In this chapter, I will introduce fifteen stretching techniques in the lay on the back (supine) position. These stretching techniques are a perfect compliment to a foot massage. Stretching techniques are combined with massage to loosen muscles quickly, and to help the client regain flexibility and a full range of motion.

The definition of stretching is "moving slightly beyond the range of motion for several seconds". Stretching properly is a delicate process: moving within the range of motion is not stretching, but we cannot push too far or we strain the muscle. The practitioner must carefully examine the limits of the natural range of motion and **stretch slightly beyond this as the client exhales.** The stretch must be applied during the exhale, because muscles are only relaxed during exhalation. A stretch should not last any longer than a few seconds, or the length of one full exhale. Some old stretching techniques teach that a muscle should be stretched for up to 30 seconds. This method does the muscle more harm than good. Never stretch a muscle past the duration of the exhale, or for longer than ten seconds. **Stretching must be applied cautiously — overstretching can result in muscle pulls or strains.**

Some of the stretching techniques shown in this chapter also loosen portions of the leg, such as the achilles tendon and calf muscles. Many of the muscles of the foot are connected to the legs, and most foot movements involve the leg muscles. Many Zoku Shin Do practitioners massage not just the foot but the entire leg as well, while some even massage the thigh and hip because the pelvis, legs, and feet are so closely connected. The Japanese word, Zoku, refers to the entire leg, not just to the foot. Full techniques for massaging the legs and hips are explained in the book *ANMA: The Art of Japanese Massage*.

Japanese Foot Massage Techniques - Example #46

Stretch the Feet Up

Japanese name of this technique

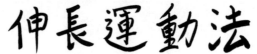

Shin Cho Un Do Ho

The purpose of this technique

Help improve the flexibility of the foot and ankle (ankle dorsal flexion)

Where it is applied on the feet

Entire feet

About this technique

Start stretching the foot with this technique to help improve the upward flexibility movement of the entire foot (ankle dorsal flexion). This technique is not used for extension of the toes, and should not apply pressure to the toes. It is very important for the foot to be relaxed while you stretch it. Make sure that the foot is properly warmed with massage techniques before you begin to stretch.

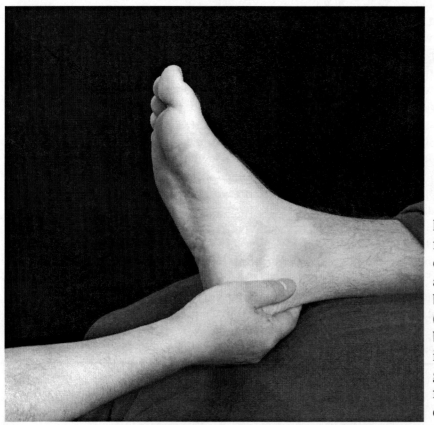

1 Grasp the heel with your inner (right) hand so that the index finger is behind the outside (lateral) ankle and the thumb is behind the inside (medial) ankle. The base of the thumb, index, and middle fingers should have a firm grip on the edge of the heel pad.

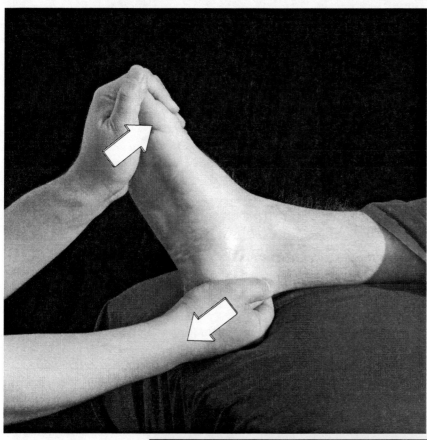

2 Squeeze with the palm of your inner hand, using just enough pressure to stabilize the heel. Gently wrap the outer (left) hand around the toes so that the heel of the palm hooks just below the ball of the foot. Have your client take a deep breath, then slowly exhale. As soon as the exhale begins, start stretching the foot by using the outer hand to push the ball of the foot away from you. At the same time, pull the heel slightly toward you with the inner hand.

3 As you stretch the foot, the toes can bend slightly backward, but **do not put pressure on the toes** to avoid hyperextension. Release and straighten the fingers of your inner hand, keeping the palm hooked to the ball of the foot. Extend the stretch slightly beyond the range of motion for the foot. Hold for about five seconds or until the end of the exhale, then release. Repeat several times, stretching slightly further each time with slightly greater pressure.

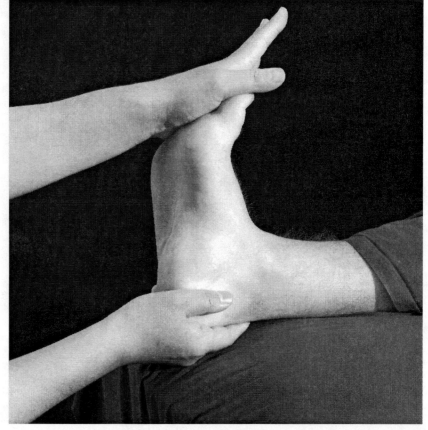

Japanese Foot Massage Techniques - Example #47

Stretch the Feet Down

Japanese name of this technique

伸長運動法

Shin Cho Un Do Ho

The purpose of this technique

Help improve the flexibility of the foot and ankle (ankle plantar flexion)

Where it is applied on the feet

Entire feet

About this technique

This example is another technique for stretching the foot, and is similar to the previous technique. The foot stretches in the opposite direction to help increase the downward flexibility movement of the entire foot (ankle plantar flexion). This will also help to stretch the muscles around the shin, and the top (dorsal) of the foot, involved in raising the foot and toes upward (dorsal flexion of the ankle).

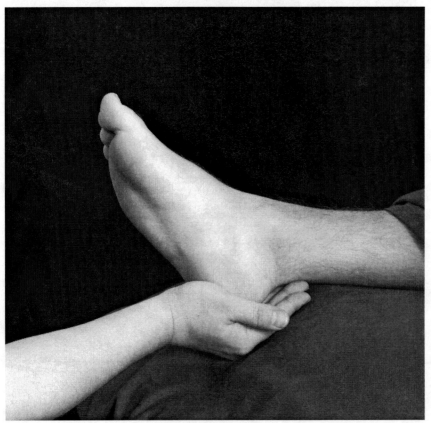

1 Place the back of the heel in the center of the palm of your inner (right) hand. Firmly grip the heel of the hand to the heel of the foot to stabilize the foot. Make sure that you do not hyperextend the wrist.

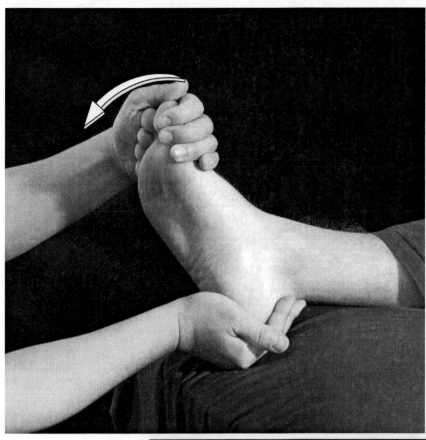

2 Grasp the top (dorsal) of the foot with your outer (left) hand. Wrap the fingers around the inside (medial) edge of the foot, and firmly grip the outside (lateral) edge with the ball of the thumb (thenar). Gently pull the top of the foot toward you as far as it will comfortably move. Have the client take a deep breath. As the exhale begins, apply pressure to bring the top of the foot further toward you, stretching the foot slightly past the comfort range.

3 As you continue to pull the top of the foot toward you, keep the heel of the inner hand pushed against the heel of the foot for support. Keep pressure to the toes minimized, **do not hyperflex the toes** by applying too much pressure. Hold for about five seconds or until the end of the exhale, then release. Repeat several times, stretching slightly further each time with slightly greater pressure.

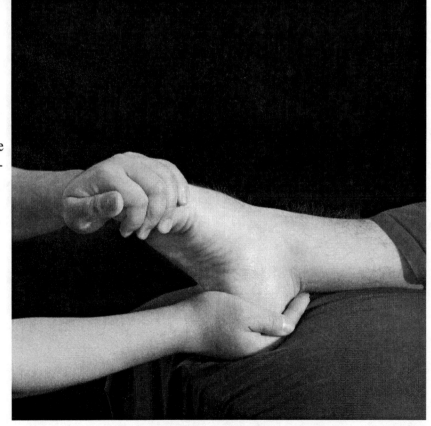

Japanese Foot Massage Techniques - Example #48

Stretch the Feet Inward

Japanese name of this technique

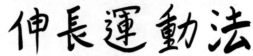

Shin Cho Un Do Ho

The purpose of this technique

Help improve the flexibility of the foot (inversion of the foot)

Where it is applied on the feet

Entire feet

About this technique

These next two examples stretch the muscles in the middle of the foot by rotating the foot both inward and outward. This example stretches the foot inward. The ability to rotate the foot inward (inversion of the foot) is one of the essential keys to proper alignment of the body structure and the ability to stabilize the balance of the body. The client does not usually feel much of a stretch, just pressure. If the client feels pain during this procedure, you can omit this technique.

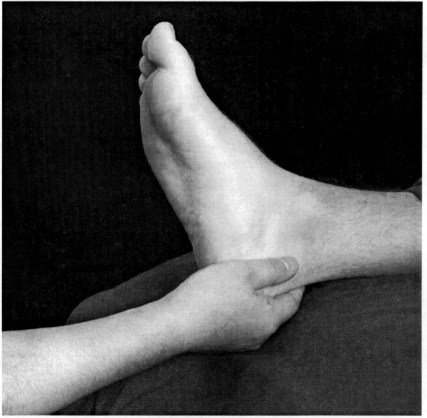

1 Grasp the heel with your inner (right) hand so that the base of the thumb, index, and middle fingers have a firm grip on both sides of the heel pad. The index finger should be behind the outside (lateral) ankle and the thumb behind the inside (medial) ankle.

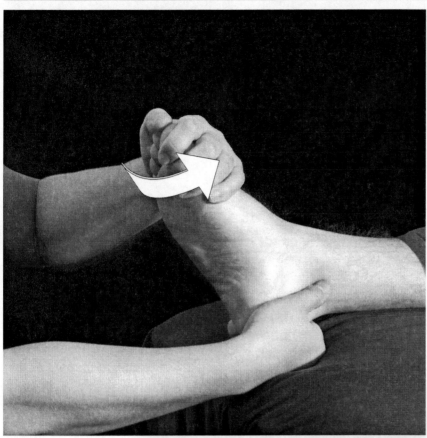

2 Grasp the toes and top (dorsal) of the foot with the outer (left) hand so that the tips of the fingers wrap around the big toe. The fingertips must maintain a firm grip on the inner (medial) side of the ball of the foot by the big toe while the heel of the hand firmly contacts the top of the foot by the fifth toe. Pull the inner side of the foot away from you with your fingertips to rotate the top of the foot. At the same time, push with the heel of the inner hand to firmly stablize the heel of the foot.

3 Gently push into the top of the foot by the fifth toe using the heel of the outer hand. The pressure of the outer hand should primarily be to the top of the foot, **do not put pressure on the toes.** Apply pressure slightly beyond the range of motion for the foot. Hold for about five seconds or until the end of the exhale, then release. Repeat several times, stretching slightly further each time with slightly greater pressure.

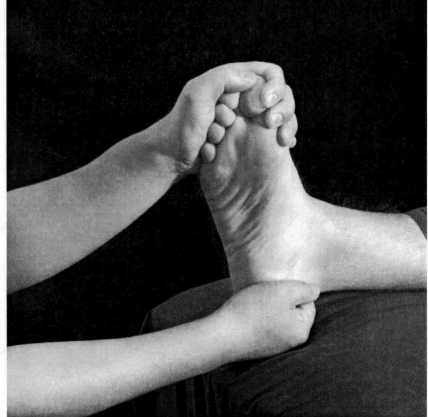

Japanese Foot Massage Techniques - Example #49

Stretch the Feet Outward

Japanese name of this technique

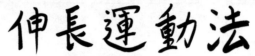

Shin Cho Un Do Ho

The purpose of this technique

Help improve the flexibility of the foot (eversion of the foot)

Where it is applied on the feet

Entire feet

About this technique

This example stretches the muscles to help improve the flexibility of the foot by rotating the foot outward. It is the companion stretch to the previous example. This stretch usually moves very little, which is normal for the range of motion of the foot, yet it is important to stretch the foot outward. A firm grip on the foot is essential for the success of this technique, but be careful not to squeeze so hard that it causes the client pain. The stretch must be effective, but not forceful.

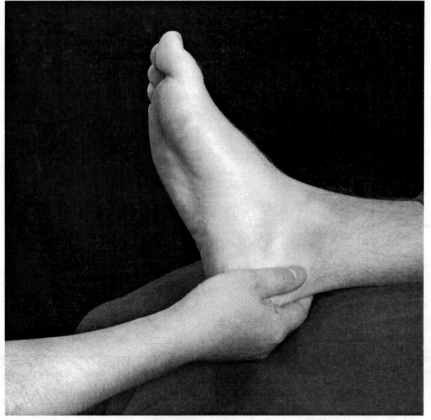

1 Grasp the heel with your inner (right) hand, placing the index finger behind the outside (lateral) ankle and the thumb behind the inside (medial) ankle. The base of the thumb, index and middle fingers should have a firm grip on both sides of the heel pad.

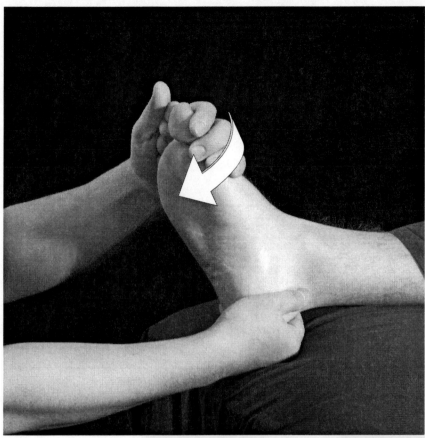

2 Grasp the top (dorsal) of the foot with the outer (left) hand so that the tips of the fingers wrap around the inner (medial) edge. The outer (lateral) edge of the foot by the fifth toe should firmly contact the outer hand just above the ball of the thumb. Rotate the inner edge of the foot toward you with the fingers of the outer hand while pressing the outer edge away from you with the ball of the thumb. The inner hand can slightly rotate in the opposite direction to help stretch the foot.

3 Continue rotating the outer side of the foot away from you. The pressure of the outer hand should primarily be against the edges of the foot. Apply pressure slightly beyond the range of motion for the foot. Minimize pressure to the toes. Hold for about five seconds or until the end of the exhale, then release. Repeat several times, stretching slightly further each time with slightly greater pressure.

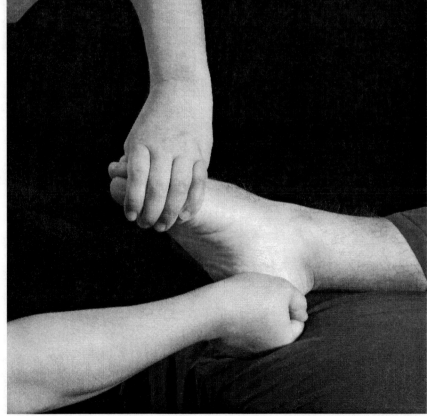

Japanese Foot Massage Techniques - Example #50

Stretch the Balls of the Feet Outward

Japanese name of this technique

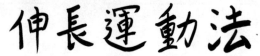

伸長運動法

Shin Cho Un Do Ho

The purpose of this technique

Stretch the ball of the foot and help restore the transverse arch

Where it is applied on the feet

Balls of the feet, over the metatarsophalangeal joints

About this technique

This example stretches the muscles and fascia in the ball of the foot by applying pressure to push outward from the center of the foot with the balls of the thumbs (radial carpal ball). This movement flattens the arch of the toes (transverse arch). Use no lubrication for this example, unless dryness of the skin inhibits sliding the balls of the thumb, because good gripping strength is essential to a good stretch.

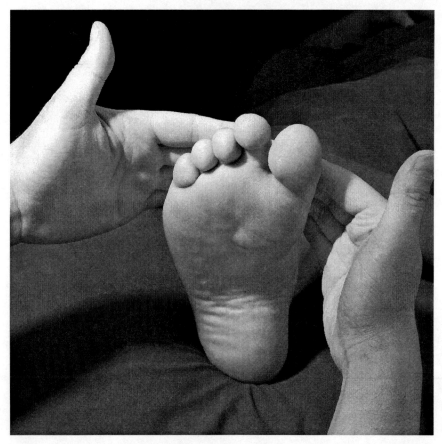

1 Place the fingers of both hands on the top (dorsal) of the foot. The fingertips should meet directly over the third foot bone (metatarsal).

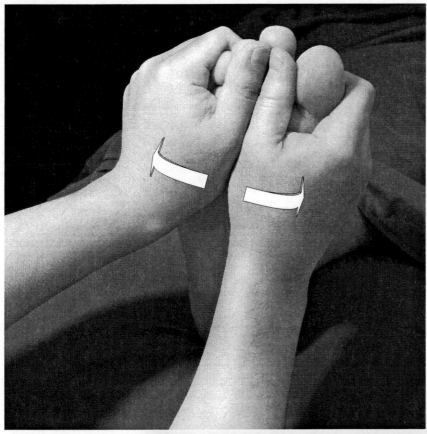

2 Wrap the palms of both hands around the foot so that the balls of the thumbs meet at the center of the ball of the foot. Apply strong pressure with the balls of the thumbs into the foot. The fingertips should provide support by pressing against the top of the foot. Maintain strong pressure to provide firm traction against the ball of the foot. Slowly separate the balls of the thumbs, moving them toward the outside edges of the foot.

3 As the balls of thumbs slide across the ball of the foot, push the fingertips into the top of the foot using them as a pivot. This straightens the arch of the toes (transverse arch) by stretching the ball of the foot. Maintain firm pressure with the fingertips to the top of the foot, but not so much pressure that it becomes painful. Release pressure once the thumbs reach the outside edges of the foot. Repeat several times on the ball of the foot, then repeat on the other foot.

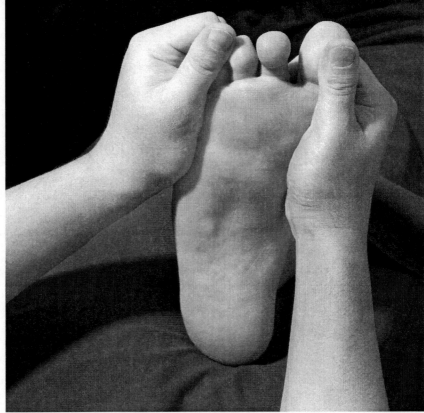

Japanese Foot Massage Techniques - Example #51

Diagonally Stretch the Balls of the Feet Outward

Japanese name of this technique

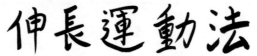

Shin Cho Un Do Ho

The purpose of this technique

Reduce tensions of the muscles and tendons by stretching the ball of the foot

Where it is applied on the feet

The balls of the feet over the metatarsals

About this technique

This example is similar to the previous one, except that the stretching is applied diagonally instead of straight outward to the sides. The foot stretches less in this technique, but it helps to increase flexibility in the ball of the foot. As with the previous example, use no lubrication unless needed. Do not overextend your wrists during performance of this technique.

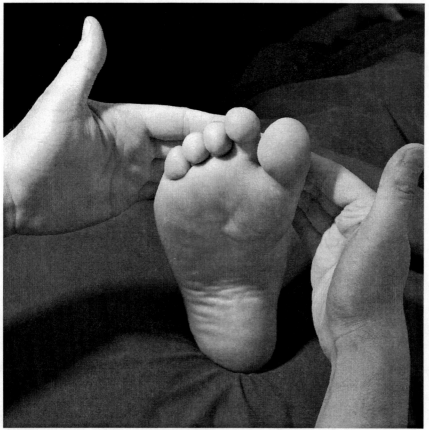

1 Use the same starting position as the previous example, placing your fingers on the top (dorsal) of the foot. Rotate the angle of the hands to the foot as needed for each step.

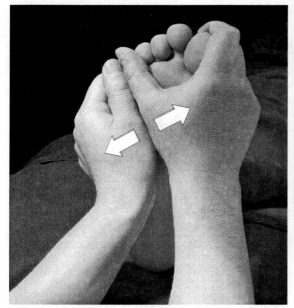

2 Place the balls (thenars) of the thumbs on the center of the ball of the foot at a 45° angle outward to the foot bones (metatarsals). Apply firm pressure between the fingertips and thumbs. Start slowly sliding the inner (right) hand toward the big toe and the outer (left) hand toward the outer (lateral) side of the foot.

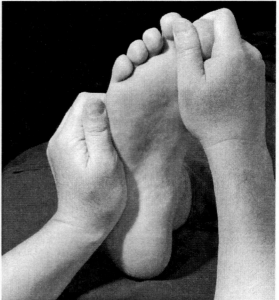

3 Stretch the ball of the foot by using your fingertips as leverage against the top of the foot. As the thumbs slide outward, apply pressure with the fingers to help straighten the arch of the toes (transverse arch). Stop when the balls of the thumbs reach the edges of the foot. Repeat several times.

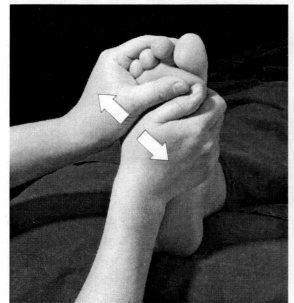

4 This is similar to Steps 2 - 3 except the balls of the thumbs are placed at a 45° angle inward to the foot bones. Start slowly sliding the outer (left) hand toward the fifth toe and the inner (right) hand toward the inner (medial) side of the foot.

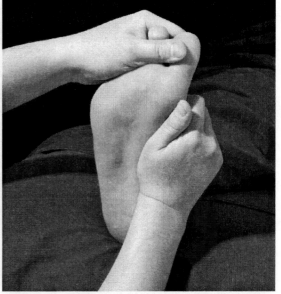

5 This variation stretches less than the previous one. Make sure you stretch slowly, using firm pressure. You can alternate between the two variations several times to maximize the stretch. Repeat on the other foot.

Japanese Foot Massage Techniques - Example #52

Stretching the Middles of the Feet Outward

Japanese name of this technique

伸長運動法

Shin Cho Un Do Ho

The purpose of this technique

Stretch the middle of the foot

Where it is applied on the feet

In the middle of the feet

About this technique

This technique is the same as Example #50, except that it is applied in the middle of the foot rather than around the ball of the foot. It stretches the muscles in the middle of the foot by pulling the sides of the foot outward. Use slow movements while the client is exhaling. Again, use no lubrication for this example unlees needed, because good gripping strength is essential to a good stretch.

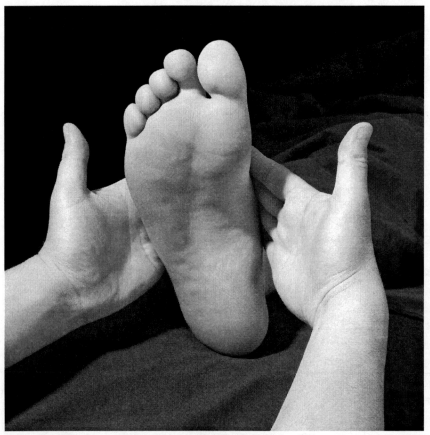

1 Place the fingers of both hands on the top (dorsal) of the foot, directly over the third foot bone (metatarsal). It is similar to the starting position of Example #50, except that the hands are further down toward the ankle, with both pinkies touching the base of the leg where it meets the foot.

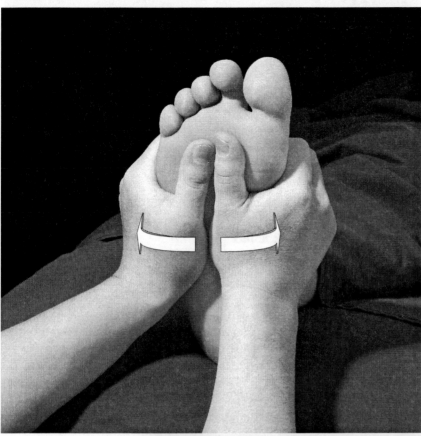

2 Wrap the palms of both hands around the foot so that the balls of the thumbs meet at the center of the middle of the foot. The tips of the thumbs should meet at the ball of the foot. Apply strong pressure with the balls of the thumbs into the foot. The fingertips become a pivot point to stretch by pressing against the top of the foot. Maintain strong pressure to assist with traction. Stretch by slowly separating the balls of the thumbs, moving them toward the outside edges.

3 As the thumbs slide outward toward the edges, maintain pressure with the fingertips. The top of the foot will push into the fingertips, stretching the middle of the foot. Release pressure once the thumbs reach the sides of the foot. Make sure that there is no stress to your wrists during the application. Repeat several times on the middle of the foot, then repeat on the other foot.

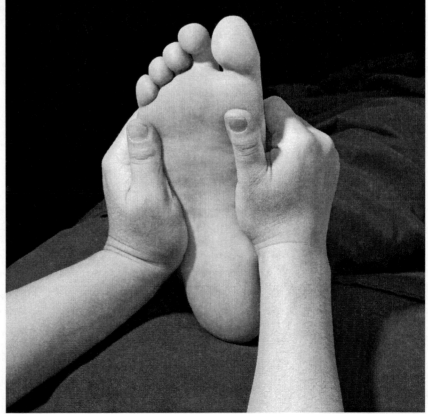

Japanese Foot Massage Techniques - Example #53

Stretching the Middles of the Feet with Thumbs

Japanese name of this technique

伸長運動法

Shin Cho Un Do Ho

The purpose of this technique

Help release dysfunctions of the fascia on the middle of the foot

Where it is applied on the feet

Middle of the feet in between the balls of the feet and the toes

About this technique

This technique uses a similar concept to steps 4 - 5 of Example #18, but this stretches the fascia and muscles instead of stroking. It is applied with much stronger pressure and uses slower movement to stretch the tissue in the middle of the foot, instead of stroking over the skin. Do not use any lubrication because a firm, strong grip to the skin is essential for this technique. Remove any existing lubricant before beginning.

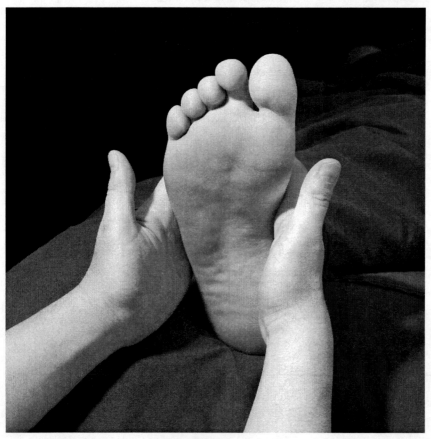

1 Place the fingers of the inner (right) hand over the first and second foot bones (metatarsals). Place the fingers of the outer (left) hand over the fourth and fifth foot bones. It is similar to the starting position of the previous technique, except that the fingers are not meeting in the center of the foot, and the hands wrap further around the sides of the foot.

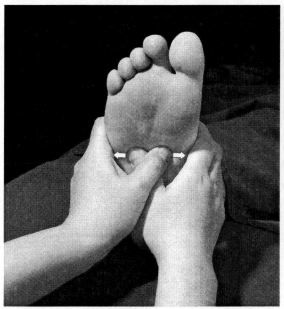

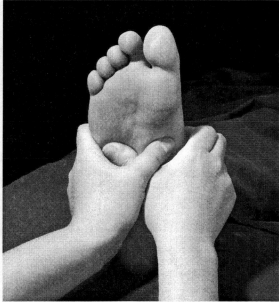

2 Cross your thumbs and place the tip of the inner thumb between the third and fourth foot bones, and the tip of the outer thumb between the second and third foot bones just below the ball of the foot. Apply firm pressure into the foot and slowly slide toward the edges.

3 Stop sliding as the thumbs reach the first and fifth foot bones. Repeat 2 - 3 times. It is important that the thumbs are kept completely straight during this entire procedure. If you feel any stress to your thumbs, you must adjust the angle to minimize the stress.

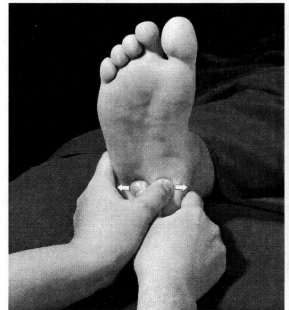

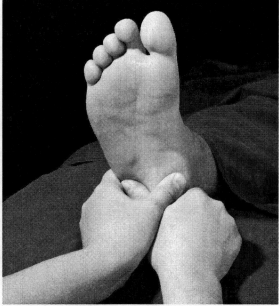

4 As you continue stretching, move down about one thumb-width at a time and repeat 2 - 3 times. As you move closer to the heel, the distance will become shorter, and harder to stretch. It is recommended that you maintain firm pressure and keep the sliding very slow.

5 Continue stretching and moving down the foot until you have reached the top edge of the heel pad. Repeat on the other foot.

Japanese Foot Massage Techniques - Example #54

Stretch the Balls of the Feet Inward

Japanese name of this technique

伸長運動法

Shin Cho Un Do Ho

The purpose of this technique

Stretch the ball of the foot and help restore the transverse arch

Where it is applied on the feet

Balls of the feet

About this technique

This example stretches the transverse arch in the opposite direction than Technique #50 does. Both techniques are often combined, one after another, to help loosen tight muscles and ligaments on the ball of the foot, as well as helping to restore the contour of the transverse arch. The transverse arch is a small arch that follows the curvature of the toes, and is essential for the proper balance of the human body and alignment of the body structure. Make sure that you are not forcing the stretch.

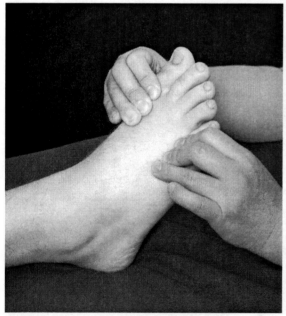

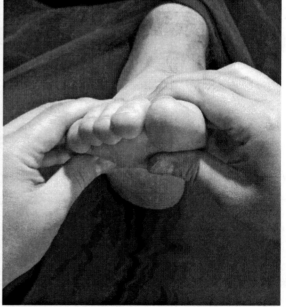

1 Place the index, middle, and ring fingers of the inner (right) hand between the first and second foot bones (metatarsals), and the index, middle, and ring fingers of the outer (left) hand between the fourth and fifth foot bones.

2 Place the thumb of the inner hand on the ball of the foot under the big toe, and the thumb of the outer hand on the ball of the foot under the fifth toe. Bring your hands and thumbs to a 90° angle to the foot by raising your elbows.

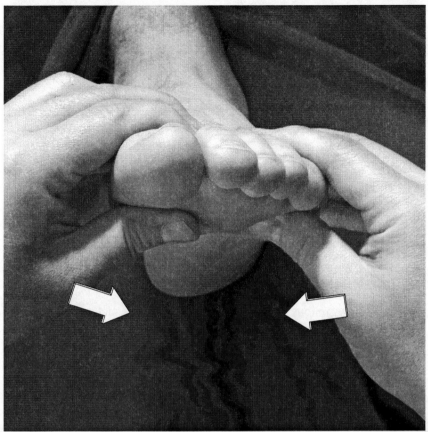

3 Apply firm, even pressure to the foot between your thumbs and fingers. Have the client take a deep breath. As the exhale begins, bring the balls of the thumbs toward each other to stretch the foot, using the tips of the thumbs as leverage. Keep the thumbs completely straight, but do not move or slide the thumbs across the foot. Your fingertips must be firmly gripped to the foot bones and pulling toward the outside egdes of the foot to assist the stretch.

4 Finish stretching as the balls of your thumbs touch each other, unless the foot is so inflexible that it is unable to stretch that far. Stretch the foot slightly beyond the range of motion. Repeat several times while adjusting your placement of the thumbs to stretch slightly different regions and increase the effectiveness of the stretching.

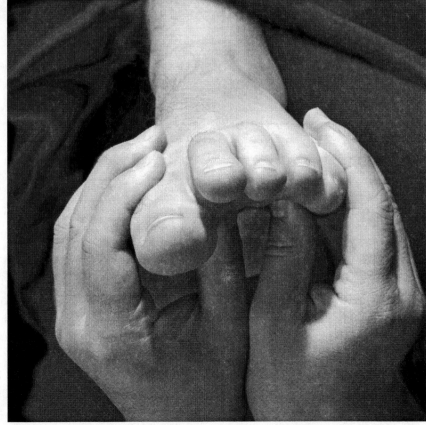

Japanese Foot Massage Techniques - Example #55

Stretch Between Each Metatarsal and Phalange

Japanese name of this technique

他動運動法

Ta Do Un Do Ho

The purpose of this technique

Increase the flexibility between the metatarsals and phalanges

Where it is applied on the feet

Between the metatarsals and phalanges in the middle of the feet

About this technique

This technique stretches between each set of metatarsals and phalanges individually to increase flexibility between them, and to help reduce muscle tension. This technique can be easily combined with other techniques that work on the ball of the foot to effectively loosen tightness over this region. As you move between the smaller toes, the foot will usually stretch less, but it is still important to stretch.

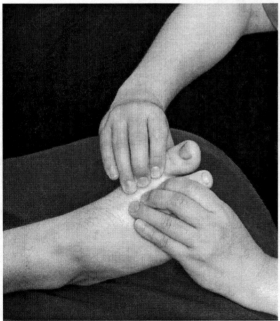

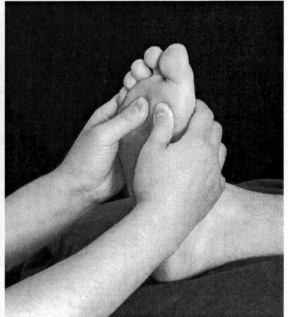

1 Place the index, middle, and ring fingers of the inner (right) hand together on the outside (lateral) edge of first foot bone (metatarsal and phalanges). Place the index, middle, and ring fingers of the outer (left) hand on the inside (medial) edge of second foot bone.

2 Place the thumb of the inner hand on the ball of the foot under the big toe and place the thumb of the outer hand on the ball of the foot under the second toe. It is very important that the thumbs remain completely straight during the entire procedure.

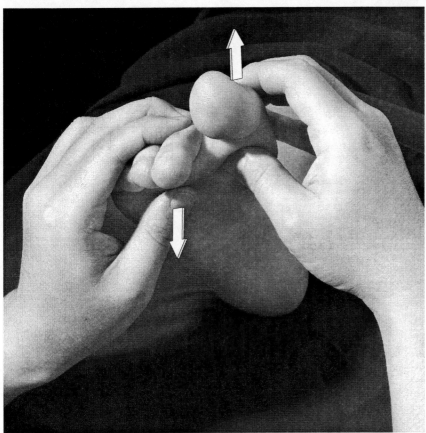

3 Apply firm pressure between the thumbs and the fingers of both hands. Push the thumb of the inner hand upward while pulling the fingers of outer hand downward. Make sure that the thumb of outer hand and the fingers of the inner hand are still gripped firmly to the foot bone for support. Do not apply any pressure to the toes.

4 As you reach the end of the range of motion, stretch the foot in the opposite direction by pushing the thumb of the outer hand upward while pulling the fingers of the inner hand downward. Repeat 6 - 10 times to loosen between the foot bones, stretching slightly further each time.

5 Repeat the same movement between each set of foot bones until you have finished between the fourth and fifth set of foot bones.

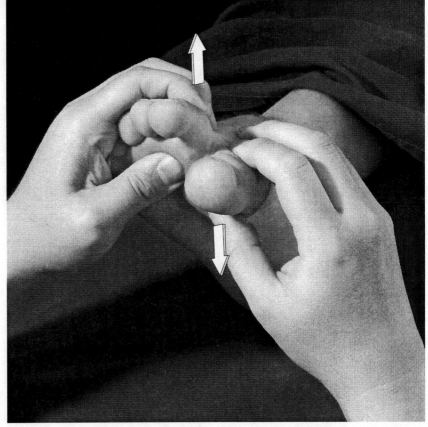

Stretch the Toes (longitudinally)

Japanese name of this technique

伸長運動法

Shin Cho Un Do Ho

The purpose of this technique

Stretch the toes longitudinally

Where it is applied on the feet

On the toes

About this technique

This and the next two examples show methods to stretch the toes. This example is used to gently stretch each toe longitudinally. Toes are a very important part of the foot, especially for the feet to properly support the body's structure and movement. If there is lubrication left on the toes, this techniques can be difficult to apply. You can wrap the toes with a sheet or towel and grasp over it for traction to make it easier.

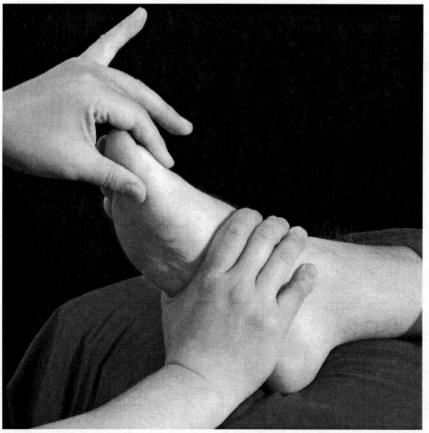

1 Grasp the foot with your inner (right) hand to firmly support and stabilize it. Grasp the big toe with the thumb, index, and middle fingers of the outer (left) hand so that the entire length of the toe is covered. The index and middle fingers should be on the top (dorsal) of the toe and the thumb on the bottom (plantar) side. Make sure that you support the big toe with the flat parts, and not the tips, of the fingers and thumbs.

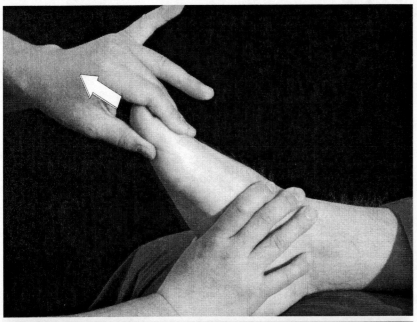

2 Stretch the big toe away from the heel (longitudinally), by pulling with your outer thumb and fingers while the inner hand slightly pushes down the foot. Apply the minimal amount of pressure needed to maintain firm traction on the toe, but not so much pressure that it is painful to the client. The movement itself is very small. Hold for 3 - 5 seconds then release.

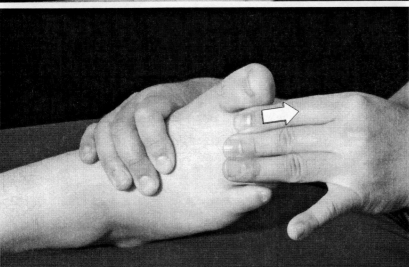

3 Move to the second toe and repeat. As the toes get narrower, it is best to grasp by the flat part of only the thumb and index finger. The entire second toe should be supported by the flats of the thumb and index finger so that the tips are touching the base of the toe.

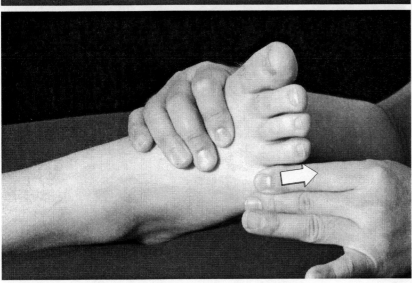

4 Continue stretching as you move down the foot toward the smallest toe. For better traction on the smaller toes, you can place your middle finger on top of the index finger for added support, but use less pressure when you pull. Repeat on the other foot.

Stretch the Toes (extension)

Japanese name of this technique

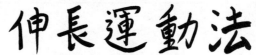

Shin Cho Un Do Ho

The purpose of this technique

Increase range of motion of the toes (with extension movement of proximal interphalangeal joints)

Where it is applied on the feet

On the toes

About this technique

This the second example of stretching the toes. Compared to the previous example, this technique requires a little more caution. There are a few ways to stretch the toe with extension movements. Many people grip the foot with one hand, placing the other hand on the bottom of the toes to stretch from there. This method is much safer and does not overextend the joints at the very tips of the toes (distal interphalangeal joints).

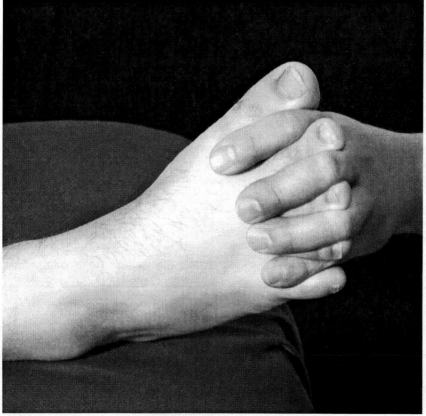

1 Interlace the fingers of your outer (left) hand through the toes, so that the tips of the fingers rest just below the webs of the toes on the top (dorsal) of the foot. The thumb should be left to the side. In some instances where the toes are too inflexible, the client has narrow spaces between the toes, or your fingers are too wide and are difficult to place properly, it would be better to avoid this technique.

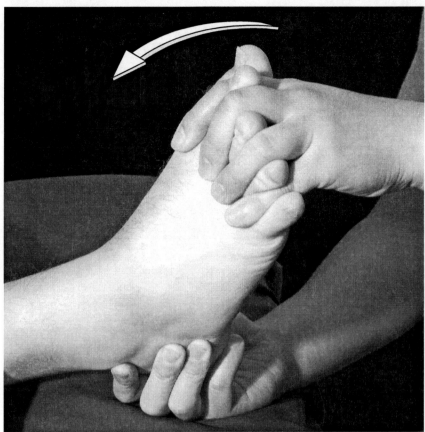

2 Place your inner (right) hand under the heel, gripping lightly with the fingers and thumb to stabilize the foot. Have your client take a deep breath. As the exhale begins, slightly bend the fingers of the outer hand at the second joint, and apply pressure to the tips of the fingers on the top (dorsal) of the foot. Using the fingers for leverage, stretch the foot away from you by bringing your elbow upward to lift the outer hand. Do not push the toes with the webs of the fingers.

3 As you stretch the toes, the foot will arch back to compensate the stretch. You must bring your elbow and hand quite high to recompensate and stretch the toes. Push slightly past the end of the range of the motion for the foot, then stop. Repeat this procedure 2 - 3 times to stretch the toes. Resetting the fingers as explained in step 1 is required for each time you stretch.

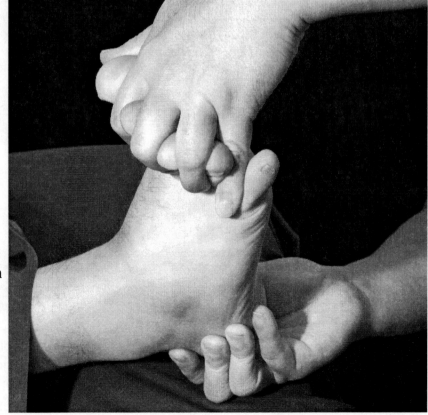

Japanese Foot Massage Techniques - Example #58

Stretch the Toes (flexion)

Japanese name of this technique

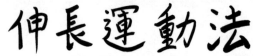

Shin Cho Un Do Ho

The purpose of this technique

Increase range of motion for the toes (with flexion movement of proximal interphalangeal joints)

Where it is applied on the feet

On the toes

About this technique

This is the third example of stretching the toes. As with the previous example, this technique must be applied with caution. The toes must be stretched far enough to be effective, but do not use excessive force. Good mobility and flexibility of the toes is important to basic human functions such as walking. Even simple movement of the toes is very essential for stabilizing and balancing the body.

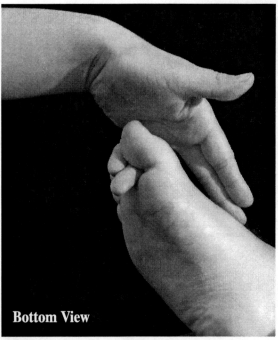

Bottom View

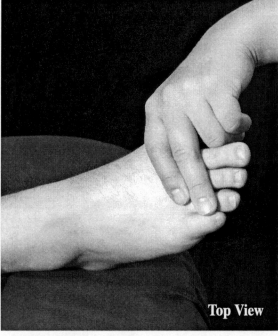

Top View

1 Place the ring and pinky fingers of your outer (left) hand between the big toe and the second toe, as shown in the Bottom View photo. Lightly place the index and middle fingers over the top (dorsal) of the foot, as shown in the Top View photo, wrapping the ring and pinky fingers around the big toe. This grip provides firm support for the toe during stretching.

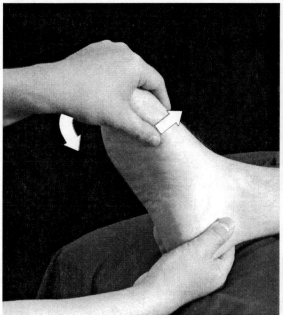

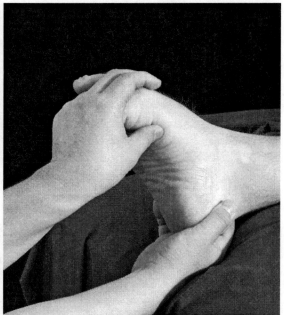

2 Place the inner (right) hand under the heel and grasp firmly for support. Place the thumb of the outer hand on the ball of the foot below the big toe. Bring the entire hand downward, using the thumb as leverage to start stretching the big toe.

3 While the client exhales, bring the foot toward you, stretching slightly beyond the end of the range of motion. The big toe must move with the index and middle fingers toward you, and should not be forced downward.

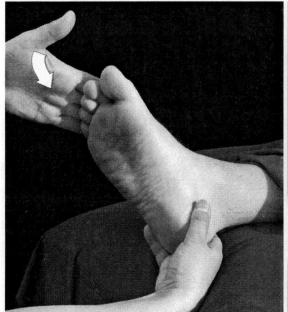

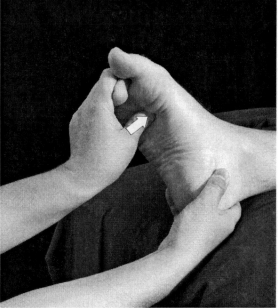

4 This is similar to steps 2 - 3, except that it is applied on the other toes. Place the fingers of the outer hand over the second through fourth toes. Gently bring the toes toward you while firmly stabilizing the heel with the inner hand.

5 If the foot is flexible enough, place the thumb of the outer hand just below the ball of the foot, using it as leverage to pull the stretch further toward you. Repeat entire procedure several times as desired.

Japanese Foot Massage Techniques - Example #59

Stretch the Achilles Tendon

Japanese name of this technique

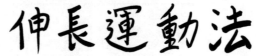

伸長運動法

Shin Cho Un Do Ho

The purpose of this technique

Reduce tension of the achilles tendon

Where it is applied on the feet

Base of the achilles tendons and the backs of the heels

About this technique

The achilles tendon is closely related to the condition of the feet, because it is the primary tendon connecting the legs to the feet. This is a good technique for reducing tension to the achilles tendon by stretching it in both directions.

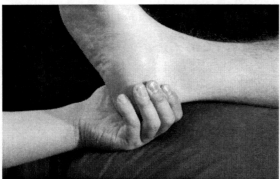

Stretching the achilles tendon inward:

1 Grasp the back of the heel with your outer (left) hand so that the heel sits in the center of the palm. Firmly hook the index, middle, and ring fingers behind the inside (medial) edge of the ankle.

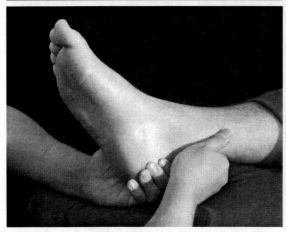

2 Hook the index, middle, and ring fingers of your inner (right) hand to the outside (lateral) of the achilles tendon. Rotate the palm of the inner hand toward the ceiling.

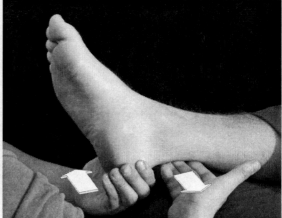

3 Stretch the achilles tendon by pulling the fingers of your inner hand inward (medially), while pulling the fingertips of the outer hand in the opposite direction to help the stretch.

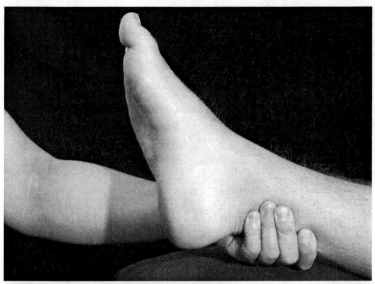

Stretching the achilles tendon outward:

4 Grasp the achilles tendon with your outer hand, so that the fingers are hooked to the inside (medial) of the achilles tendon.

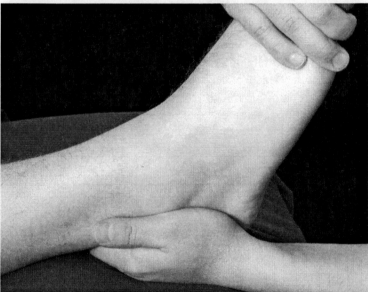

5 Grasp and stabilize the top (dorsal) of the foot around the toes with the inner hand. The heel of the hand or the ball of the thumb (thenar) should firmly contact the outside (lateral) edge of the back of the heel.

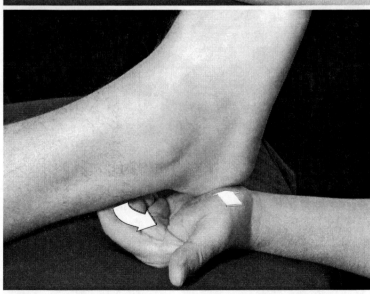

6 Stretch the achilles tendon outward (laterally) by pulling the fingers of the outer hand. At the same time, push the heel of the hand into the back edge of the heel of the foot. Rotate the outer hand, using the heel of the hand as a pivot point for the stretch. Rotation of the hand is done by moving the elbow in toward your torso, not by wrist movement alone. Make sure not to hyperextend your wrist. Repeat both stretches as desired.

Japanese Foot Massage Techniques - Example #60

Stretch the Metatarsals Down

Japanese name of this technique

伸長運動法

Shin Cho Un Do Ho

The purpose of this technique

Reduce muscle tension on the top (dorsal) of the foot

Where it is applied on the feet

On the top and bottom (dorsal and plantar) of the feet

About this technique

This the last example and has been one of my favorite foot massage and stretching techniques for a long time. This example nicely combines stretching the top of the foot and slow, deep stroking on the middle of the sole of the foot. It is the only stretching technique that requires slight lubrication. For better results, use strong pressure and stroke slowly. This technique works best when the client is exhaling during the procedure. Your shoulders, elbows, and wrists should be kept fairly relxed during this technique.

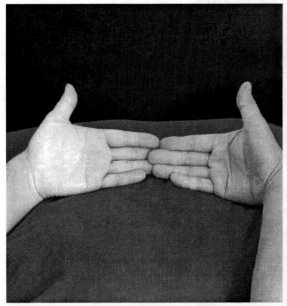 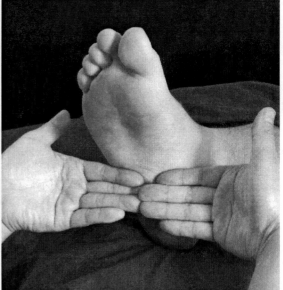

1 The index, middle, and ring fingers of both hands should point toward each other, and slightly overlap at the tips. Your thumbs should be pointed straight up, at a 90 ° angle to the fingers.

2 Maintaining the hand position in step 1, place the outside (lateral) edges of your index fingers just above the heel pad. All of the fingers should be tightly held together.

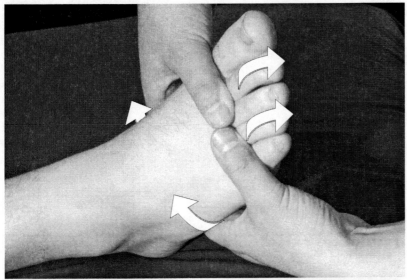

3 Place your thumbs together at the base of the toes on the top (dorsal) of the foot. Press the top of the foot downward with the thumbs, without applying pressure to the toes. Using the thumbs for leverage, push upward with the index fingers toward the ceiling. This procedure is done by dropping your forearms to rotate the wrists.

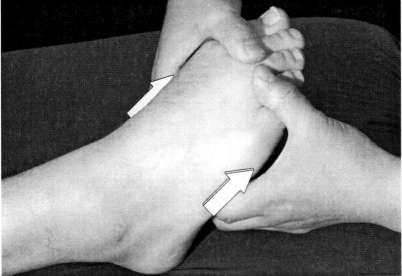

4 Slowly stroke up the foot with the index fingers toward the thumbs. Maintain firm upward pressure during the stroke using the thumbs as leverage. Make sure that the index fingers are properly supported from beneath by the other fingers.

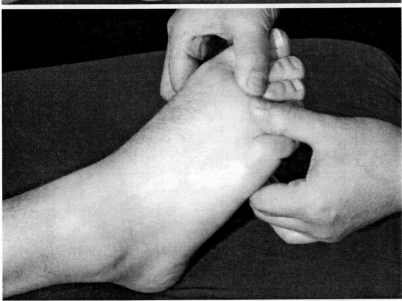

5 Stop stroking as the index fingers reach the middle of the ball of the foot. Repeat three times or as often as you desire on each foot.

Chapter Eleven

JAPANESE FOOT MASSAGE TECHNIQUES
Lay on the Stomach Position

Japanese foot massage is usually applied in either the lay on the back (supine) position as explained in the previous four chapters, or in the lay on the stomach (prone) position. Rarely are both positions used one after another in the same treatment, unless someone would require an intensive foot massage lasting longer than 20 minutes. A foot massage is usually best kept under 20 minutes because the foot is a small area and is easily overworked to the point where the client may become discomforted or extremely sensitive. Japanese foot massage is primarily part of Zoku Shin Do reflexology, which is usually performed in the lay on the back position, therefore up to this point all of the Japanese foot massage techniques have been explained in that position.

However, it is beneficial to understand how to give a foot massage in the lay on the stomach position. There may be times when people have a difficult time laying on their back, such as with a lower back injury or with other special medical conditions. It is also convenient and effective to combinefoot massage with work on the calf muscles, achilles tendons, and the backs of the legs, because they work together and effect each other.

Most of the techniques in the lay on the back position can be performed with minor modifications as the lay on the stomach position. Each position has its own advantages and disadvantages. In this chapter, I explain two positions for application of techniques in the lay on the stomach positions--from the side of the client and from the end of the table. Each of these has its own advantages and disadvantages. Also provided are a few examples to demonstrate how to transfer the techniques introduced in the previous four chapters to the lay on the stomach position.

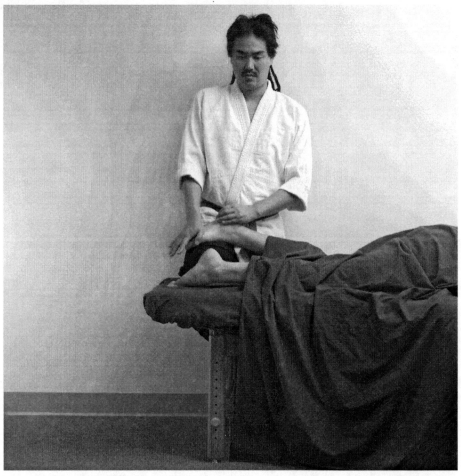

Apply on the table from the side - Lay on the stomach (Prone) position:

When working from the side position, I use my knee as support beneath the client's ankle instead of using a pillow or bolster. Using the knee allows you to move slightly up and down to adjust the position of the support as needed, which is essential for many techniques. For example, when working on the achilles tendon, you would need to move the knee slightly toward the head so that the foot moves freely. While working on the foot, you would need to move the knee down toward the toes to provide firm support beneath the foot so that you can apply deeper pressure. It also helps to stabilize your body. If you are using a table, you will usually want to place the knee closer to the client's toes. If it is difficult for you to place your knee on the table, you might substitute a bolster or pillow for support, but it will limit application of some of the techniques.

When using a massage table, it is important to have the height of the table adjusted properly, so that the knee can be comfortably placed. If the massage table is too high, your shoulders can tire more easily, and if too low, you will constantly be leaning over.

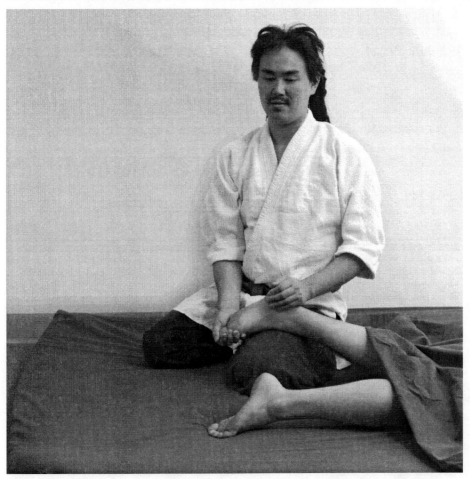

Apply on the floor from the side - Lay on the stomach (Prone) position:

If you prefer to give foot massage on the floor, or do not have a massage table, the lay on the stomach position can be easily used. Often a mat, futon, or a thick blanket is used to add cushion for comfort. You can kneel (seiza position) and place the client's ankle on top of your leg. Use the leg closest to the client's head (instead of the other as previously shown) for this position, because it minimizes body turning while applying the massage and it is easier to apply deeper pressure. The ankle should be placed on the middle of your upper leg, not too close to your torso so that the foot does not come near your genital region, but not so far down that you have to constantly be leaning over. You can substitute by using your lower leg, but it will require constant rotating of your upper torso. You can support the ankle that you are not working on for comfort.

If you have a hard time kneeling, you can sit cross-legged, but it is more difficult to apply heavy pressure and is not recommended. Generally, you will only need to maintain this position for a short time, but if needed, you can sit on a small pillow for comfort.

Application of Japanese Foot Massage -
Lay on the stomach (prone) position applied from side.

Many techniques in the previous four chapters can be easily
modified to work on the client in the lay on the stomach position.
Here are a few examples of techniques to show modifications
and adjustments for working in this position. Most of the techniques will require some modification because you will be applying from a different angle, and also because the foot and ankle
are less mobile than in the lay on the back positions.

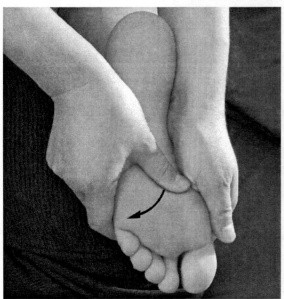 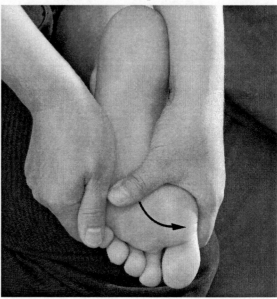

This is the same procedure as Example #6, except in the prone position. The foot is less likely to
move from left to right to support the thumb movement, so it must be applied much slower.

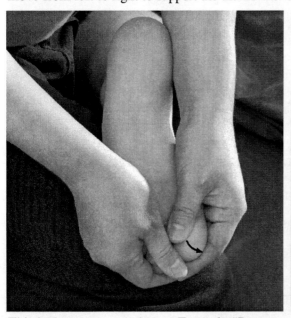 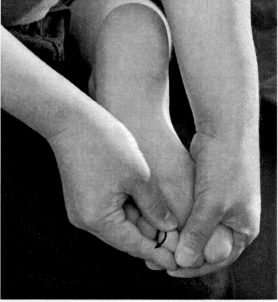

This is the same procedure as Example #7, except in the prone position. It is easier to stroke
downward instead of away from you, as it is applied in the lay on the back position.

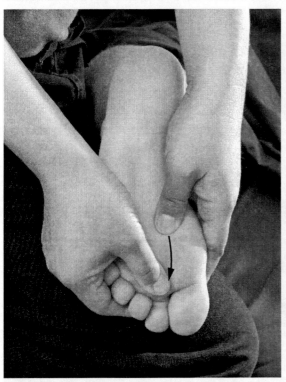 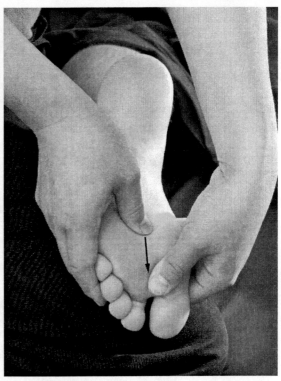

This is the same procedure as Example #17, except in the prone position. Because you can use your body weight to help with the stroke in this position, it is easier to apply deeper pressure as you stroke over the ball of the foot with alternating thumbs.

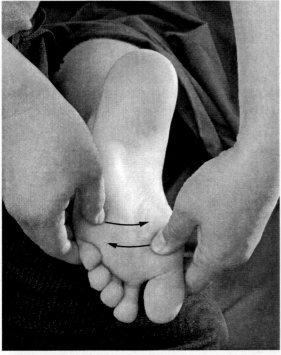 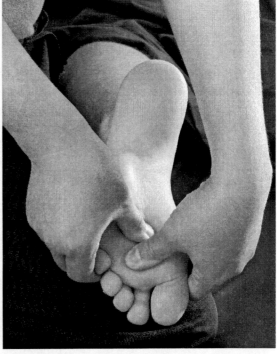

This is the same procedure as Example #18, except in the prone position. Because you can use your body weight in this position and press the foot against your knee, it is easier to apply deeper pressure as you cross-stroke over the ball of the foot with your thumbs.

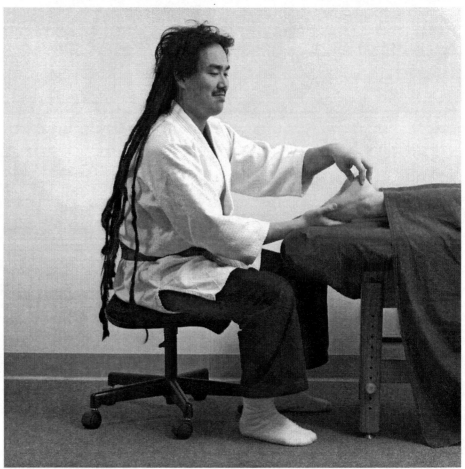

Apply on the table from the end - Lay on the stomach (Prone) position:

You can also apply massage by sitting at the end of the table by the client's feet when the client is in the lay on stomach position. Again, it is important that the height of the table and chair are properly adjusted to minimize stress to the hands and wrists, and also to help reduce tiring of your arms and shoulders. The height of the table should be comparable with the height as when applied from the side position, but adjust as needed.

The side position is excellent for applying massage to the upper half of the foot, while this position is excellent for working on the heel of the foot. The foot does not usually need any support beneath the client's ankle, unless they have an injury or a difficult time staying semi-stretched on the table. The majority of people will not have much problem without support for short periods of time, since many people sleep on the stomach without ankle support. If needed, a low pillow or bolster can be placed under the ankle for support and comfort. A large bolster or foot support might be used, but is not recommended for this position because the foot may be raised too high so that it sits at a sharper angle, making it difficult to apply massage.

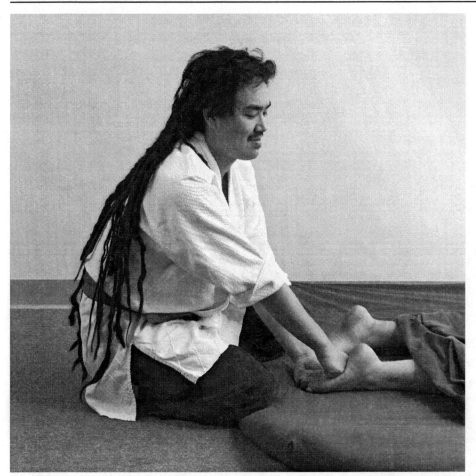

Apply on the floor from the end - Lay on the stomach (Prone) position:

When working on the floor or a mat, kneel (seiza position) at the edge of the pad. Generally, no bolster is used so that you can apply good, firm pressure into the feet. Kneeling at the feet allows you to apply pressure straight down by leaning forward with your bodyweight. Some people may find kneeling difficult, even for a short time, and if kneeling is not possible, you can sit cross-legged; if possible though, the kneeling position is best.

If the client is not comfortable without a bolster or pillow to support the ankles, it is best to firmly support entire top (dorsal) of the foot, ankle, and lower half of shin. A large foot support, such as generally used in the lay on the back positions, will also work here if needed. Do not use a round bolster for support just under the ankle because the foot will drop into a sharper angle and increase stress to your wrist. If needed, you can place support under the ankle that you are not working on for the client's comfort.

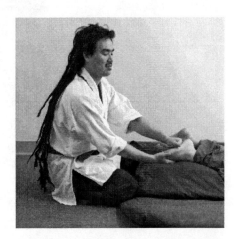

**Application of Japanese Foot Massage -
Lay on the stomach (prone) position applied from end.**

Many of the techniques in the previous four chapters can be easily applied in this position with minor modifications as demonstrated in the few examples here. This position is also excellent
for working on the heel of the foot and surrounding regions.

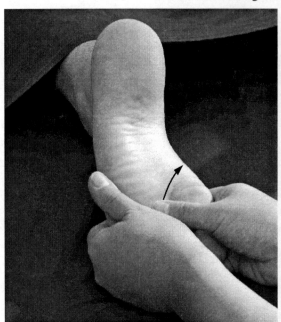 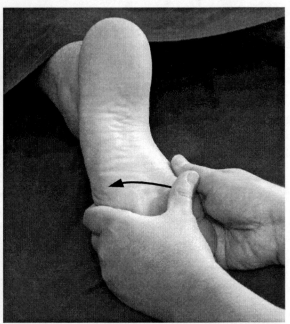

This is the same procedure as Example #6, except in the prone position. You are applying alternating thumb strokes, except the thumbs are pointing toward the heel instead of the toes.

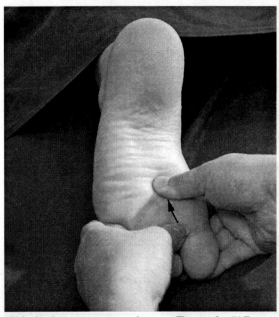 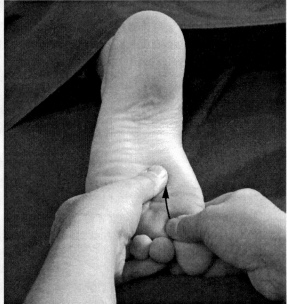

This is the same procedure as Example #17, except in the prone position. You are using alternating thumbs to stroke deeply between the metatarsals and over the balls of the feet, except you are
stroking toward the heel instead of the toes, and pushing the muscles in different directions.

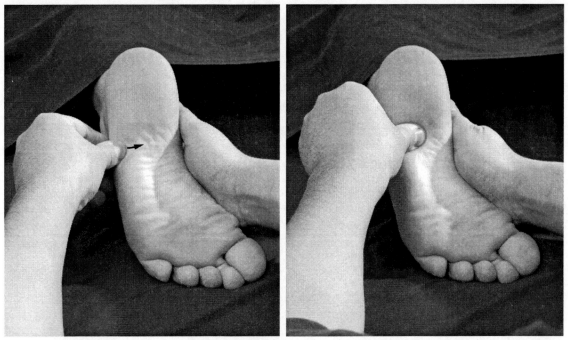

This is the same procedure as Example #26, except in the prone position. Stroke inward (medially) from the outer edge of the foot by pushing the foot with the inner hand. In this position, the foot will not move as much to support the stroking, so the thumb itself must stroke slightly to compensate. Make sure that the thumb is kept completely straight while stroking.

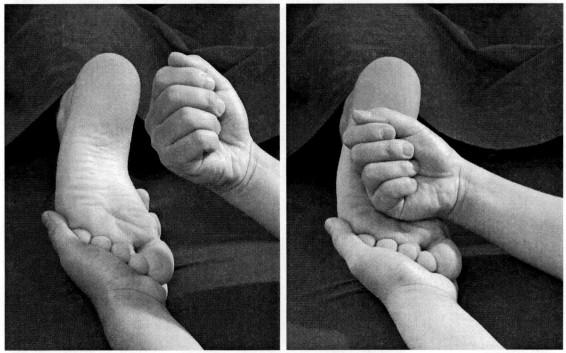

This is the same procedure as Example #41, except in the prone position. Again, a different part of the hand is used to apply percussion, so make sure that you grasp the top (dorsal) of the foot for firm support. In this position, the foot arches more, so adjust the angle of your hand to fit the contour of the foot. Again, make sure that you adjust the strength of the percussion according to the sensitivity of the client.

Chapter Twelve

AFTERWARD

A famous Japanese proverb says "Aging starts from the feet." As I explained earlier, there is a close connection between the feet and health. Japanese foot massage is a very effective method of the healing arts, not just for the feet, but for the entire body and mind as well. When applied properly, it can help to prevent many ailments and slow the aging process. As a practitioner of Japanese foot massage, it is important to be aware of the great effects massage can have. The best way to learn Japanese foot massage is to work with a partner, so you can practice and also receive massage. Receiving is a an important part of learning to understand how the foot massage feels and how each individual technique effects your body. It is also better to practice with someone who will give you honest feedback, both good and bad, so that you can develop and improve your senses for application.

One of the biggest concerns among students is determining what are the right and wrong ways to apply techniques. There is neither a right nor wrong way to perform Japanese foot massage, Zoku Shin Do, nor any other of the healing arts. It simply works or does not, and the bottom line is that you can do whatever you like, as long as you do not hurt your client or yourself. Of course, there are basic things you should not do, or are not recommended to do, to avoid harming yourself or your client. I have studied from three different masters (sensei), and each had different techniques, different reflexion concepts, different ways of diagnosis and different ways to treat the same conditions. My masters gave me good foundations, and I adapted my own ideas and experiences from many sources for over fifteen years to create my own style of Zoku Shin Do along with Japanese foot massage. The examples shown in this book come from my own personal style of Zoku Shin Do techniques which I use in my practice, and may be different from other Zoku Shin Do practitioners.

When you are giving Japanese foot massage or Zoku Shin Do, it is important that you have confidence in your work and a clear vision of what you want to achieve, rather than just applying foot massage for better circulation and comfort. It is important that when you give a massage you are comfortable and relaxed. Confidence comes from experience and experience comes from practice. If you are not confident and are nervous, your client may have a difficult time relaxing into your massage.

It is also very important that you are centered when you are giving massage. This does not mean that you are focused. You can be centered without focusing, but people often confuse the two. Centered means that you are internally, and not just physically present in a peaceful, calm condition. Certain meditations and exercises can enhance mind-centering skill, but it becomes essential as you become an advanced level practitioner of East Asian healing arts.

I have spent a tremendous amount of time and effort to best describe Japanese foot massage, but there are limitations to studying massage from a book, regardless of the number of photographs and illustrations. Since it is not possible for me to be next to all students interested in learning Japanese foot massage and East Asian foot reflexology, this book is a first step. If you are interested in more information, have any questions, comments and suggestions about any of the material covered in this book, or if you want information about times and locations of the workshops, feel free to contact:

Kotobuki Publications
attn: Mochizuki
P.O. Box 19917
Boulder, CO   80308-2917
1-800-651-2662 from within the continental U.S.
or visit our website at www.anma.com

This book is the popular edition of the foot massage portions of Zoku Shin Do, the Art of East Asian Foot Reflexology training manual. I selected all of the foundation and important techniques from that book. I plan to develop visual learning aids to supplement this book. I also plan to further develop Zoku Shin Do training text books and the popular editions of these texts may become available to the public in the future.

It is one of my goals to introduce this wonderful tradition to western countries, and my hope to contribute some closeness between family and friends in this busy and complex time. Whether you are learning Japanese foot massage for personal and family growth or to enhance professional skills as a massage therapist, acupuncturist, pedicurist, etc., I am confident that my workshops and this book will help you and all your relations to live more peacefully and harmoniously.

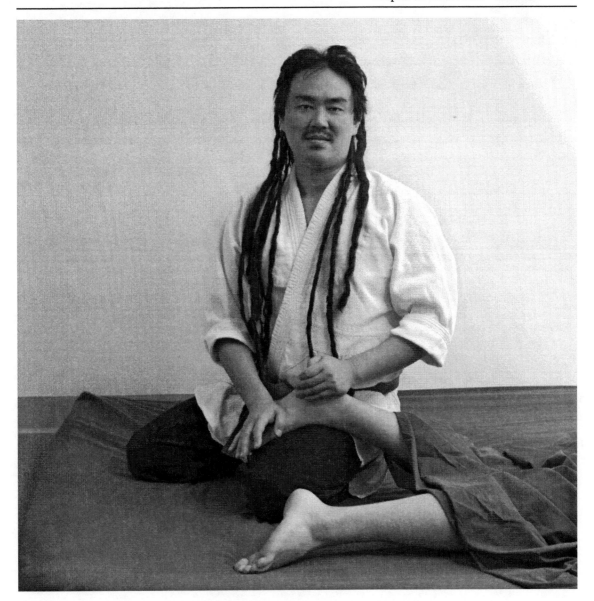

Thanks again to all those people who show interest in our way of the healing arts.

Good Health to You!

James Shogo Mochizuki

INDEX

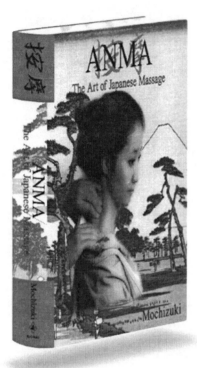

ANMA

ANMA
The Art of Japanese Massage

Anma originated in China over 4,000 years ago and was introduced to Japan about 1,300 years ago. Swedish massage and Shiatsu are among the massage forms which grew out of this rich tradition. *Anma: The Art of Japanese Massage* is the first Japanese-authored massage book published in English about Anma. Complemented with over 1000 photographs and illustrations, this text comprehensively explains the art and methods of Anma.

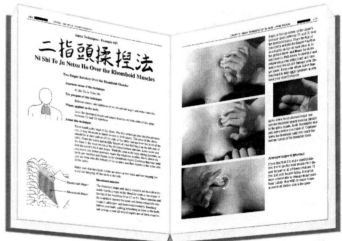

This book features:

- History and principles of Anma
- Nine Anma application techniques
- 101 application examples for the entire body
- Over 1,000 detailed photos and illustrations
- 421 pgs Softcover, ISBN 1-57615-000-3
  $ 35.^{00}

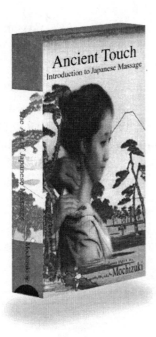

Ancient Touch
Introduction to Japanese Massage

This video is a visual demonstration of Anma Japanese massage, Japanese facial massage, and Japanese foot massage. This is your chance to preview the unique qualities of these massage forms.

This video demonstrates the nine fundamental Anma techniques, giving a good illustration of Anma application to different parts of the body.

This video also demonstrates the warm-up techniques of Japanese foot massage.

Finally, the three-stage procedures of Japanese facial massage are covered (cleansing, moisturizing, and energizing stages), and there is a demonstration of proper neck massage.

This is not an instructional video; it is a demonstrational video so that you can preview a sample of this art as performed by Sensei Mochizuki.

running time: approximately 55 minutes

ISBN 1-57615-035-6

- VHS (U.S. and Canada) $19.⁹⁵
- PAL (Europe) $22.⁹⁵

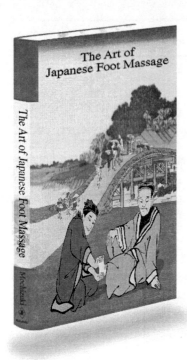

Zoku Shin Do
The Art of
East Asian Foot Reflexology
Popular Edition

Zoku Shin Do, the oldest known form of East Asian foot reflexology, originated in China over five thousand years ago. **Zoku Shin Do :The Art of East Asian Foot Reflexology** details the method of foot massage that arose from this ancient tradition. Sixty easy-to-follow examples of foot massage techniques are shown in both the supine and prone positions. This book also includes full explanations of meridians, pressure points and foot stretching techniques. Over 300 photographs and illustrations span this 223 page volume.

This book features:

- Application techniques of Japanese Foot Massage
- Brief history & principles of Zoku Shin Do
- 60 examples of applications for the Foot
- Over 300 detailed photos and illustrations
- 223 pgs Softcover, ISBN 1-57615-010-0
  $ 24.⁹⁵

Zoku Shin Do
The Art of
East Asian Foot Reflexology

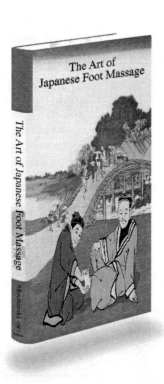

Zoku Shin Do :The Art of East Asian Foot Reflexology Instructional Video demonstrates the entire repertoire of Japanese foot massage, technique by technique. Special attention will be given to the development of sequence. This follows the instructional format of the book, designed as an adjunct to it; each procedure is taught step by step for a clear visual tutorial of every application.

- CD-ROM (U.S. and Canada)
  Macintosh compatible
  available Spring-Summer 1998

- Set of 2 Videos-(PAL only, for Europe)
  available Winter 1997

Call for price information and availability

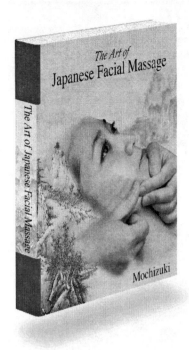

The Art of
Japanese Facial Massage
Popular Edition

Japanese Facial Massage is different from every other method of facial massage. It uniquely combines very effective methods of facial massage with traditional East Asian concepts. Fifty-five examples of techniques covering the face and neck are demonstrated throughout the three different stages of application. Over 300 photographs and illustrations supplement over 211 pages of detailed text. **The Art of Japanese Facial Massage** is the most comprehensive facial massage book ever written.

This book features:

- Application techniques of Japanese Facial Massage
- Japanese concepts of health and beauty
- 55 application examples for the face and neck
- Over 300 detailed photos and illustrations
- 211 pgs Softcover, ISBN 1-57615-025-9
  $ 24.^{95}

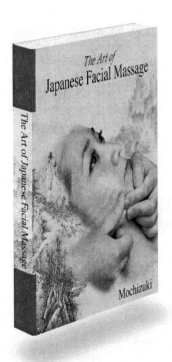

The Art of
Japanese Facial Massage

The Art of Japanese Facial Massage Instructional Video demonstrates the entire repertoire of Japanese facial massage, technique by technique. Special attention will be given to the development of sequence. This follows the instructional format of the book, designed as an adjunct to it; each procedure is taught step by step for a clear visual tutorial of every application.

- CD-ROM (U.S. and Canada)
  Macintosh compatible
  available Spring-Summer 1998
- Set of 2 Videos-(PAL only, for Europe)
  available Winter 1997

Call for price information and availability

Meridian Dolls

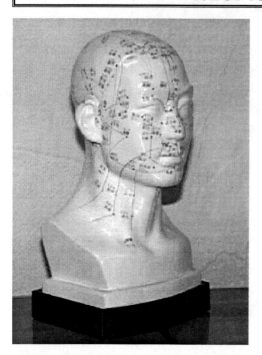

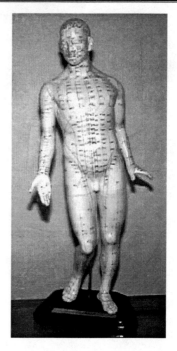

Meridian Doll, Head and Face

Approximately 8 inches high, this doll clearly illustrates the positions of all the facial and head Tsubo, as well as the meridians.
$24.⁹⁵

Meridian Doll, Full Body

Approximately 17 inches high, this doll is available in male and female models, and illustrates the entire Keiraku and Tsubo systems.
$29.⁹⁵ please specify male or female model

Posters

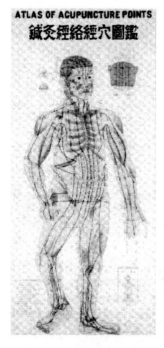

Atlas of Acupuncture Points (tsubo)

Comes as a set of two charts, front and back, 16 x 42 inches. This is an affordable chart which shows the points and meridians in a traditional format.
This chart is designed to provide a high-quality alternative to the expensive professional charts and the cheap beginners' charts.
$14.⁰⁰ set

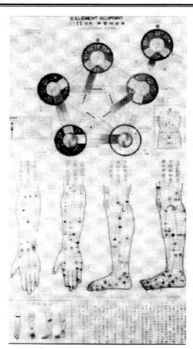

Five Element Acupuncture Chart

This is a very well-drawn and comprehensive chart. It is the only available chart to relate the Five Phases to the triple burner organ-- the San Sho.

$24.⁹⁵

Japanese Music--Compact Discs

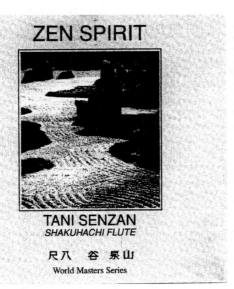

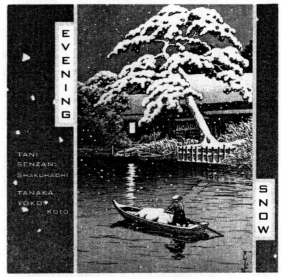

Zen Spirit

Eight traditional recordings of Shakuhachi Master
Tani Senzan. These are exquisite instrumental solos
of one of the most refined and difficult instruments
in Asian culture. The Shakuhachi flute has been
used as an adjunct to Zen meditation since the 14th
century and is deeply moving and calming music.
$15.^{95}

Evening Snow

Seven recordings by Tani Senzan and Tanaka
Yoko on the Shakuhachi and Koto, two beautiful
traditional instruments. The koto is a 13-string
zither which has been played since medieval
times. This is a combination of traditional and
modern compositions.
$15.^{95}

T-Shirts

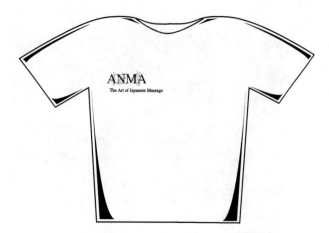

ANMA
The Art of Japanese Massage

New Anma: The Art of Japanese Massage

- 3-Color printing on the front
  - "ANMA" in black over gold calligraphy
  - "The Art of Japanese Massage" in red
  2-Color printing on the sleeve
  - "Japanese Massage & Bodywork Institute" in red and black

- 100% Fruit of the Loom Heavyweight Cotton

- Sizes: M, L, XL or XXL available

- Colors: White, Natural (Unbleached), Sage (Blue-green), Burgundy, and Purple

- Prices:
  $14.^{00} (any sizes)

How To Order

Two easy ways to order:

Order by phone

Call toll free **1-800-651-2662** (International 303-442-6161)
Mon-Fri 9:00am - 5:00pm, Sat 9:00am - 12 noon MST
Order with CREDIT CARDS ONLY Visa-Mastercard-Discover accepted

Order by mail

mail in your completed order form with check, money order or credit card info to:

Kotobuki Publications
P.O. Box 19917
Boulder, CO 80308-2917

Make check or money order payable to KOTOBUKI PUBLICATIONS, (U.S. funds only)
or fill out credit card information.
For faster service, money order or credit card payment is suggested.

Kotobuki Publications

Boulder, Colorado
1-800-651-2662

Order Form

Ordered By:

Name _____

Address _____

_____

City _____ State/Prov. _____

Zip/Postal Code _____ Country _____

Phone _____
(Just in case of questions on your order)

Ship to: (Only if different from "Ordered By")

Name _____

Address _____

_____

City _____ State/Prov. _____

Zip/Postal Code _____ Country _____

All prices are subject to change,
Please call 1-800-651-2662
for further information.

ITEM #	QTY	DESCRIPTIONS	PRICE /EACH	TOTAL
000		ANMA : The Art of Japanese Massage (Book)	$35.00	
035		Ancient Touch : Introduction to Japanese Massage (Video)	$19.95	
010		The Art of Japanese Foot Massage Popular Edition (Book)	$24.95	
020		The Art of Japanese Facial Massage Popular Edition (Book)	$24.95	
D-02		Meridian Doll, Head and Face	$24.95	
D-01		Meridian Doll, Full Body circle choice: Male, Female	$29.95	
P-02		Atlas of Acupuncture Points (Posters)	$14.00	
P-01		Five Elements Acupuncture Chart (Poster)	$24.95	
CD-03		Zen Spirit (Music-CD)	$15.95	
CD-04		Evening Snow (Music-CD)	$15.95	
CT-01		ANMA T-shirts circle choice: M, L, XL, or XXL wh, nat, sag, bur, pur	$14.00	

METHOD OF PAYMENT:

☐ VISA ☐ Master Card ☐ Discover ☐ Check/M.O.

Card No.
☐☐☐☐☐☐☐☐☐☐☐☐☐☐☐☐

Exp.Date
☐☐☐☐ Your Signature _____

MERCHANDICE TOTAL	
SALES TAX (CO deliveries only)	
SHIPPING (per order)	$4.95
TOTAL	

Thank You!
Kotobuki Publications